Pediatric Urology

Editor

CARLOS R. ESTRADA JR.

UROLOGIC CLINICS OF NORTH AMERICA

www.urologic.theclinics.com

Consulting Editor
KEVIN R. LOUGHLIN

August 2023 • Volume 50 • Number 3

ELSEVIER

1600 John F. Kennedy Boulevard • Suite 1800 • Philadelphia, Pennsylvania, 19103-2899

http://www.theclinics.com

UROLOGIC CLINICS OF NORTH AMERICA Volume 50, Number 3
August 2023 ISSN 0094-0143, ISBN-13: 978-0-443-18413-0

Editor: Kerry Holland
Developmental Editor: Malvika Shah

Urologic Clinics of North America (ISSN 0094-0143) is published quarterly by Elsevier Inc., 360 Park Avenue South, New York, NY 10010-1710. Months of issue are February, May, August, and November. Business and Editorial Offices: 1600 John F. Kennedy Blvd., Suite 1800, Philadelphia, PA 19103-2899. Periodicals postage paid at New York, NY and additional mailing offices. Subscription prices are $415.00 per year (US individuals), $832.00 per year (US institutions), $100.00 per year (US students and residents), $473.00 per year (Canadian individuals), $1040.00 per year (Canadian institutions), $100.00 per year (Canadian students/residents), $546.00 per year (foreign individuals), $1040.00 per year (foreign institutions), and $240.00 per year (foreign students/residents). Foreign air speed delivery is included in all *Clinics* subscription prices. All prices are subject to change without notice. **POSTMASTER:** Send address changes to *Urologic Clinics of North America*, Elsevier Health Sciences Division, Subscription Customer Service, 3251 Riverport Lane, Maryland Heights, MO 63043. **Customer Service: 1-800-654-2452 (US). From outside the United States, call 1-314-447-8871. Fax: 1-314-447-8029. E-mail: JournalsCustomerServiceusa@elsevier.com (for print support)** and **JournalsOnlineSupport-usa@elsevier.com (for online support)**.

Reprints. For copies of 100 or more, of articles in this publication, please contact the Commercial Reprints Department, Elsevier Inc., 360 Park Avenue South, New York, New York 10010-1710. Tel.: 212-633-3874; Fax: 212-633-3820; E-mail: reprints@elsevier.com.

Urologic Clinics of North America is covered in MEDLINE/PubMed (*Index Medicus*), *Excerpta Medica, Current Contents/Clinical Medicine, Science Citation Index,* and *ISI/BIOMED.*

Contributors

CONSULTING EDITOR

KEVIN R. LOUGHLIN, MD, MBA
Emeritus Professor of Surgery (Urology),
Harvard Medical School, Visiting Scientist,
Vascular Biology Research Program at Boston
Children's Hospital, Boston, Massachusetts,
USA

EDITOR

CARLOS R. ESTRADA JR, MD, MBA
Urologist-in-Chief, Boston Children's Hospital,
Department of Urology, Associate Professor of
Surgery, Harvard Medical School, Boston,
Massachusetts, USA

AUTHORS

JOSEPH BORER, MD
Department of Urology, Boston Children's
Hospital, Associate Professor, Department of
Surgery (Urology), Harvard Medical School,
Boston, Massachusetts, USA

ERIC M. BORTNICK, MD
Pediatric Urology Fellow, Department of
Pediatric Urology, Boston Children's Hospital,
Boston, Massachusetts, USA

NICOL BUSH, MD, MCS
Hypospadias Specialty Center, The Colony,
Texas, USA

PETER Y. CAI, MD
Urology Fellow, Department of Urology,
Boston Children's Hospital, Boston,
Massachusetts, USA

CHING MAN CARMEN TONG, DO
Department of Pediatric Urology, The
University of Alabama at Birmingham,
Birmingham, Alabama, USA

RAJEEV CHAUDHRY, MD
Assistant Professor of Urology, University of
Pittsburgh Medical Center, Children's Hospital
of Pittsburgh, Pittsburgh, Pennsylvania, USA

EMILY R. CHEDRAWE, MD
Division of Pediatric Urology, IWK Health
Centre, Department of Urology, Dalhousie
University, Halifax, Nova Scotia, Canada

EARL Y. CHENG, MD
Division of Urology, Ann & Robert H. Lurie
Children's Hospital of Chicago, Department of
Urology, Northwestern University Feinberg
School of Medicine, Chicago, Illinois, USA

NICHOLAS G. COST, MD
Associate Professor, Division of Urology,
Department of Surgery, University of Colorado
School of Medicine, Surgical Oncology
Program, Children's Hospital Colorado,
Aurora, Colorado, USA

JONATHAN S. ELLISON, MD
Department of Urology, Medical College of
Wisconsin, Children's Hospital of Wisconsin,
Milwaukee, Wisconsin, USA

EMILIE K. JOHNSON, MD, MPH, FACS
Division of Urology, Ann & Robert H. Lurie
Children's Hospital of Chicago, Department of
Urology, Northwestern University Feinberg
School of Medicine, Chicago, Illinois, USA

DANIEL T. KEEFE, MD, MSc
Division of Urology, IWK Health Centre,
Department of Urology, Dalhousie University,
Halifax, Nova Scotia, Canada

MICHAEL P. KURTZ, MD, MPH
Assistant Professor of Surgery, Boston
Children's Hospital, Harvard Medical School,
Boston, Massachusetts, USA

RICHARD S. LEE, MD
Associate Professor, Department of Surgery,
Harvard Medical School, Department of
Urology, Boston Children's Hospital, Boston,
Massachusetts, USA

TED LEE, MD, MSc
Department of Urology, Boston Children's
Hospital, Boston, Massachusetts, USA

CALEB P. NELSON, MD, MPH
Associate Professor of Surgery, Department of
Pediatric Urology, Pediatrics, Harvard Medical
School, Boston Children's Hospital, Boston,
Massachusetts, USA

HANS G. POHL, MD
Professor, Urology and Pediatrics, The George
Washington University School of Medicine and
Health Sciences, Urology, Children's National
Hospital, Washington, DC, USA

RODRIGO L.P. ROMAO, MD, MSc
Assistant Professor, Departments of Surgery
and Urology, Divisions of Urology and Pediatric
Surgery, IWK Health Centre, Dalhousie
University, Halifax, Nova Scotia, Canada

AMANDA F. SALTZMAN, MD
Associate Professor, Department of Urology,
University of Kentucky, Lexington, Kentucky,
USA

WARREN SNODGRASS, MD
Hypospadias Specialty Center, The Colony,
Texas, USA

GREGORY E. TASIAN, MD, MSc, MSCE
Division of Urology, Department of Surgery,
Children's Hospital of Philadelphia,
Philadelphia, Pennsylvania, USA

JAX WHITEHEAD, MD
Division of Endocrinology, Ann & Robert H.
Lurie Children's Hospital of Chicago,
Department of Pediatrics, Northwestern
University Feinberg School of Medicine,
Chicago, Illinois, USA

JOHN S. WIENER, MD
Professor of Urology and Pediatrics,
Department of Urology, Duke University
Medical Center, Durham, North Carolina, USA

Contents

Fetal upper tract urinary system dilation is one of the most common findings on prenatal ultrasonography. Rarely, this may represent fetal lower urinary tract obstruction (LUTO), of which posterior urethral valves are the predominant etiology. LUTO is the most dire fetal urologic diagnosis, as it affects not only the baby's management after birth but sometimes the course of the pregnancy itself. A variety of treatment options are available prenatally; these include observation, vesicoamniotic shunt placement, amnioinfusion, and attempts at direct treatment of the valves themselves. All fetal interventions carry substantial risks; caution should attend every discussion of treatment.

Congenital hydronephrosis can be classified and managed based on the Urinary Tract Dilation consensus scoring system. Ureteropelvic junction obstruction is one of the most common causes of hydronephrosis in the pediatric population. Although most cases can be managed conservatively with follow-up and serial imaging, some patients need surgical repair because of renal function deterioration, infections, or symptoms. Additional research to create predictive algorithms or develop noninvasive biomarkers for renal deterioration is necessary to better identify surgical candidates. The robotic-assisted approach for pyeloplasty is becoming increasingly widespread and associated with shorter hospital stay, high success rates, and low complication rates.

A ureterocele is a congenital cystic dilatation of the intravesical ureter that may affect either a single system kidney or the upper pole of a duplex system. The position of ureteral orifice correlates with function of associated renal moiety. Ureteroceles associated with good renal function and prompt drainage or ureteroceles associated with no renal function can be managed nonoperatively. Endoscopic puncture of ureteroceles addresses most cases; iatrogenic reflux may rarely require secondary surgery. Robot-assisted laparoscopic upper pole nephroureterectomy and ureteroureterostomy procedures are rarely associated with complications.

Although investigations over the past 2 decades have improved our understanding of the natural history of vesicoureteral reflux (VUR) and helped identify those at higher risk of both VUR itself as well as its potential severe sequelae, debate exists regarding key aspects of care, including when to perform diagnostic imaging and which patients benefit from continuous antibiotic prophylaxis. Artificial intelligence and machine learning have the potential to distill large volumes of granular data into practical tools that clinicians can use to guide diagnosis and management decisions. Surgical treatment, when indicated, remains highly effective and is associated with low morbidity.

Exstrophy-epispadias complex encompasses a spectrum of disorders with lower abdominal midline malformations, including epispadias, bladder exstrophy, and cloacal exstrophy, also known as Omphalocele–Exstrophy–Imperforate Anus–Spinal Anomalies Complex. In this review, the authors discuss the epidemiology, embryologic cause, prenatal findings, phenotypic characteristics, and management strategies of these 3 conditions. The primary focus is to summarize outcomes pertaining to each condition.

Neurogenic lower urinary tract dysfunction (NLUTD) remains a formidable challenge to pediatric urologists to achieve the goals of renal preservation and the reduction of urinary tract infections as well as the attainment of continence and independence as children grow toward adulthood. Tremendous progress has occurred over the past 50 years which have witnessed an evolution in focus from mere survival to optimal quality of life. This review presents four separate guidelines for the medical and surgical care of pediatric NLUTD, most commonly related to spina bifida, to highlight the change in approach from expectant to more proactive management.

Differences of sex development (DSD) encompass a broad range of conditions in which the development of chromosomal, gonadal, or anatomic sex is not typically male or female. Terms used to describe DSD are controversial, and continuously evolving. An individualized, multidisciplinary approach is key to both the diagnosis and management of DSD. Recent advances in DSD care include expanded genetic testing options, a more nuanced approach to gonadal management, and an emphasis on shared decision-making, particularly related to external genital surgical procedures. The timing of DSD surgery is currently being questioned and debated in both medical and advocacy/activism spheres.

UROLOGIC CLINICS OF NORTH AMERICA

SERIES OF RELATED INTEREST
Surgical Clinics of North America
https://www.surgical.theclinics.com/

Foreword

July 1, 1982: The Birth of the Modern Urology Service at Boston Children's Hospital

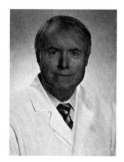

Kevin R. Loughlin, MD, MBA
Consulting Editor

It was the middle of June in 1982, and I received a phone call from the urology administrator at Brigham and Women's Hospital, who told me that Dr Ben Gittes wanted to see me in his office that day at 6 PM. This was before the era of e-mails, so the direct phone call made it seem even more ominous. I quickly went through my mental checklist: op notes and discharge summaries up to date, Wednesday night conferences seemed to be going well as had morbidity and mortality conferences. Nonetheless, I arrived that night at the meeting with some trepidation. Was I in trouble?

I entered his office, and Dr Gittes motioned to a chair in front of his desk and said, "Have a seat, Kevin." He then began," As you know, Hardy Hendren is coming over to Children's from MGH on July 1. He and Alan both have strong egos, but they both know that it is in everyone's interest to make this work. I am going to have you start there as chief resident at Children's in July. Your job is to make sure everything goes smoothly and to keep everyone happy. Understand?" The three chief residents in my year were Lionel Fraser, Gerry Andriole, and me. I considered it a compliment that Ben had chosen me to start at Children's, but that didn't mitigate my anxiety as July 1 approached.

A few days after my meeting with Ben, Alan Retik took me out to dinner. He explained his expectations to me. All of Dr Hendren's urology patients would be on the urology service, and their

surgeries would be covered by urology residents. I was fortunate that summer to have the opportunity to work with two outstanding fellows, Jay Vacanti of pediatric surgery and Tony Casale of pediatric urology, who made my job easier than it might have been.

Dr Retik and Dr Hendren couldn't have been nicer to me. My apprehension at the beginning of July soon dissolved into wonder as each day was filled with fascinating cases in the operating room. When my rotation concluded at the end of October, I was disappointed that it was over. It had been a wonderful 4 months. The entire Children's staff—nurses, techs, residents, and fellows, were great, and everyone had worked together in harmony. I remember the radiology conferences run by Dr Bob Lebowitz, which just enhanced the surgical experience even more.

As they say, the rest is history. The summer of 1982 began, what I consider, the birth of the "modern era" of Boston Children's Urology. It became a regional, national, and international resource for urologic training and research. It is a credit to both Ds Retik and Hendren that they laid the foundation for the ongoing excellence of the Boston Children's Hospital urology service.

Since 1982, there have been 59 clinical fellows, 14 research fellows, and several hundred urology residents who have trained at Boston Children's Hospital. It remains a shared resource for the five urology residency programs in greater Boston. Many of those who trained at Boston Children's

Urol Clin N Am 50 (2023) ix–x
https://doi.org/10.1016/j.ucl.2023.05.002
0094-0143/23/© 2023 Published by Elsevier Inc.

urologic.theclinics.com

Hospital have gone on to outstanding academic careers of their own.

There are currently 17 full-time clinical urology attendings and three full-time research urology attendings. Current extramural research funding is in the millions of dollars. In the past four decades there have been three urology chiefs: Alan Retik, David Diamond, and Carlos Estrada. This issue of *Urologic Clinics*, edited by Dr Estrada, illustrates the growth of knowledge and advances in technique that have occurred in pediatric urology over the past decades. The diverse authorship in this issue reflects the multiple hospitals where progress has paralleled the advances witnessed at Boston Children's Hospital.

It was once said that a society can be judged by how it cares for its most vulnerable—its children and its elderly. That is one of the reasons that makes urology sui generis. In my view, I can say that I think pediatric urologists represent the best in us. Their diagnostic acumen and surgical skill are the hallmarks of our specialty. Dr Estrada has assembled world-renowned experts to contribute to this issue. He and his colleagues have produced an issue that is a filling legacy to the underpinning provided by Drs Retik and Hendren, which began decades ago.

Kevin R. Loughlin, MD, MBA
Visiting Scientist
Vascular Biology Research Program at
Boston Children's Hospital
300 Longwood Avenue
Boston, MA 02115, USA

E-mail address:
kloughlin@partners.org

Preface
Pediatric Urology 2023

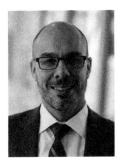

Carlos R. Estrada Jr, MD, MBA
Editor

In the 5 years since the last pediatric urology-focused *Urologic Clinics* was published, the world has changed significantly. The global COVID-19 pandemic cost more than one million Americans their lives and forced an almost complete halting of the care of our patients for a few long and dark months. American politics are as polarized as ever, and profound differences in beliefs are increasingly affecting how we manage pediatric patients, particularly those with differences in sexual development and gender dysphoria. With these challenges swirling around us, our specialty remains steadfastly committed to the betterment of pediatric lives and tackling challenges that we have faced since the beginning of our specialty, namely, preservation of renal function, surgical correction of the common and complex urologic congenital problems, and management of pediatric urologic cancer. Advances in surgery, particularly in robotics, minimally invasive surgery, and miniaturization of endoscopic instruments, have brought new, innovative, and exciting solutions to these ongoing clinical challenges.

In this issue of the *Urologic Clinics*, an esteemed group of pediatric urologists present the most up-to-date information on topics that form the core of pediatric urology. These are broadly grouped into problems related to (1) urinary tract obstruction and vesicoureteral reflux, including those diagnosed prenatally, ureteropelvic junction obstruction, ureterocele, and primary reflux; (2) congenital differences that are associated with the biggest challenges and controversies in our specialty, including epispadias-exstrophy complex, neurogenic lower urinary tract dysfunction, differences in sex development, and hypospadias; (3) pediatric urologic cancer; and (4) common problems in pediatric urology, including pediatric urolithiasis and undescended testis. I anticipate that the reader will greatly enjoy the wonderful content and leave with an updated understanding of pediatric urology in 2023.

I would like to thank the authors for their hard work and commitment to academic pediatric urology. I am privileged to call them colleagues and grateful for their willingness to contribute to this issue.

Carlos R. Estrada Jr, MD, MBA
Boston Children's Hospital
Department of Urology
300 Longwood, Avenue HU350, Boston, MA
02445, USA

E-mail address:
carlos.estrada@childrens.harvard.edu

Urol Clin N Am 50 (2023) xi
https://doi.org/10.1016/j.ucl.2023.05.001
0094-0143/23/© 2023 Published by Elsevier Inc.

Prenatal Diagnoses and Intervention

Michael P. Kurtz, MD, MPH

KEYWORDS

- Posterior urethral valves • LUTO • Fetal intervention • Hydronephrosis • Obstruction
- Pediatric urology

KEY POINTS

- The ideal candidate for fetal intervention for lower urinary tract obstruction (LUTO) is a singleton male fetus, normal karyotype, with the clear diagnosis of LUTO with the onset of anhydramnios at 20 weeks gestation.
- Fetal intervention carries substantial risks to the pregnancy and the fetus postnatally.
- A trial of serial amnioinfusion is ongoing; the bilateral renal agenesis subgroup has shown concerning results.

INTRODUCTION

Treatment of congenital urologic anomalies has always been at the forefront of fetal intervention. Fetal surgery began in 1963 with the transfusion of blood,[1] followed by exchange transfusions in 1964. Any form of fetal surgery was exceptionally hazardous at this point, and intervention before birth remained a quiet field for nearly 2 decades. Then, in 1982, an 18-year-old G1P0 woman presented at 20 weeks gestation with severe oligohydramnios.[2] Ultrasound had only recently acquired sufficient resolution to make this diagnosis securely. On vesicocentesis, 95 mL of urine was aspirated from the fetal bladder, indicating severe lower urinary tract obstruction (LUTO). At 21 weeks gestation, Dr Michael Harrison and colleagues at the University of California, San Francisco performed an open hysterotomy. Twenty-five minutes later they had completed bilateral open ureterostomies and returned the fetus to the womb. Postoperatively the mother recovered and returned home for an uneventful 3 months. At 35 weeks contractions began, and the baby was born 2 days later. Maximum respiratory support was unable to oxygenate the infant and care was withdrawn after 9 hours. In concluding his New England Journal of Medicine report, Dr Harrison wrote "innovative fetal treatment must be fully tested in the laboratory, carefully considered in light of current diagnostic and therapeutic uncertainties, honestly presented to the mother, and family, undertaken only with great trepidation." This advice was prescient; the triumphs and failures of fetal therapy for LUTO remain largely unchanged 4 decades later.

ETIOLOGY AND CLASSIFICATION

The primary differential diagnosis of LUTO in the male fetus is between posterior urethral valves (PUVs) and urethral atresia. There are several less common causes, including Prune belly syndrome (also called Eagle-Barrett syndrome and triad syndrome), which includes abdominal wall muscular deficiency and undescended testes in additional to urinary system abnormalities (classically a large bladder and dilated distal ureters). The bladder outlet may also be obstructed by anterior urethral valves, a prolapsed ureterocele, or other urethral abnormalities, the latter two of which have

The authors confirm no commercial or financial conflicts of interest.
Boston Children's Hospital, Harvard Medical School, 300 Longwood Avenue, Hunnewell 390, Boston, MA 02115, USA
E-mail address: michael.kurtz@childrens.harvard.edu

Urol Clin N Am 50 (2023) 351–359
https://doi.org/10.1016/j.ucl.2023.04.006

condition-specific fetal interventions which will be discussed later. Bladder outlet obstruction may also result from a genitourinary sinus and massive hydrocolpos, but fortunately these often have distinct imaging findings other than the dilated bladder itself.

Classification of LUTO has recently been clarified with acceptance of the Ruano system. This separates cases into three stages. Stage I represents mild LUTO with normal amniotic fluid index (AFI), normal renal echogenicity with absence of cysts and dysplasia, and a favorable urinary chemistry on bladder aspiration (if performed). No intervention is indicated, and observation is important. Serial ultrasounds may detect if there is a change in amniotic fluid, or if findings suggesting renal disease become more prominent. Most maternal-fetal medicine specialists perform ultrasounds approximately at 2-week intervals for this condition. Stage II LUTO includes cases of oligohydramnios or anhydramnios with hyperechoic kidneys but absent cystic changes. With favorable urinary chemistry, intervention may be indicated. This is the stage of most importance for fetal surgeons, as most of the cases arise from this cohort. Stage III is severe LUTO with abnormal renal function and unfavorable ultrasound findings; here, the role of intervention is stated to be less clear.[3] In these cases, observation alone may be appropriate. As some will progress to in utero renal failure, a vesicoamniotic shunt may fail to restore amniotic fluid volume. A final stage was added later, Stage IV, and this "in utero renal failure" group represents a distinct cohort with the most severe disease.[4] Management here is purely expectant.

As both urethral atresia and PUV may present with posterior urethral dilation, it is not possible to determine the diagnosis with complete confidence prenatally. The diagnosis is only secured definitively with attempts at urethral catheterization and fluoroscopy for babies after birth. Just recently a group form the Netherlands published a prospective cohort of cases using bladder size to help define this precise problem.[5] The investigators constructed nomograms of two measures of fetal bladder size: the longitudinal bladder diameter and ultrasonographic determination of fetal bladder volume. The bladder diameter was measured in the precise midsagittal plane, and it is important to note that this is measured at the inner border of the bladder wall at the dome and the inner border at the bladder neck. This is a wise selection, as sonographically the difference in echogenicity of fluid and tissue is the most consistent interface at which to place a caliper. LUTO cases often have profoundly thickened bladder walls, larger than the width of small bowel, and so in this case we are not measuring the size of the bladder but rather the volume of the bladder's fluid contents. They assessed these parameters in 225 pregnancies with 1238 measurements obtained. Both PUV and urethral atresia cases showed dramatically increased bladder sizes, as expected, but the urethral atresia cases had longitudinal bladder measurements than twofold higher on average. The cohort size was generous with 76 cases of PUV and 22 cases of urethral atresia. Using this, a Z-score cutoff was determined of 5.2; this yielded 74% sensitivity and 86% specificity in discerning PUV from urethra atresia. While it fits with clinical experience that larger bladders are more common in urethra atresia, this intriguing findings deserves validation in a separate center.

FETAL INTERVENTION
Vesicoamniotic Shunt

Harrison and Rocket shunts are small extruded plastic tubes built in the style of a double-J stent, and first brought to market in the 1980s (**Table 1**). Because of their design, the internal lumen is around 3Fr or smaller, and they are prone to clogging and dislodgement; around half of shunts will require replacement due to malfunction or dislodgement.[6] Despite this, the PLUTO trial showed in an as-treated analysis that the relative risk with respect survival was far higher in the treated arm at 28 days (RR 3.20, $P = .03$), 1 year (RR 4.27 $P = .02$), and 2 years (RR 4.27, $P = .02$).[7] Although there are numerous criticisms of the trial, including an approximately 15% crossover, the unselected nature of LUTO cases, under-recruitment, and the heterogeneity in interventional volume across centers, this signal is strong and suggests that there is likely benefit to intervention in some cases of LUTO. The evidence for this is not as strong as hoped at trial onset.[8] Given the dislodgement, an additional shunt has come to market in Europe. Researchers Bonn and Cologne recently published their experience comparing a silicone Somatex shunt versus Harrison hunts. Here, 36.4% of the Somatex shunts dislodged, which was dramatically superior to the 87.5% dislodgement rate of the Harrison shunt[9] but still leaves substantial room for improvement. Shunting remains risky. Even with newer technology preterm premature rupture of membranes (PPROM) occurred in 1/9 cases (affected fetus was not viable), and of the 6 that survived to term, all had chronic kidney disease (CKD), and one did not survive beyond the neonatal intensive care unit (NICU).[10]

Table 1
Fetal intervention

	Benefits	Risks
LUTO due to presumed PUV or urethral atresia		
Shunt placement	Agnostic of LUTO etiology, restore amniotic fluid volume, best studied LUTO intervention	Chorioamnionitis, chorioamniotic membrane separation, PPROM, fetal urinary ascites, shunt dislodgement/need for repeat shunt placement, abdominal wall defect, visceral injury
Fetal cystoscopic treatment	Potential for definitive treatment of the obstruction, restore amniotic fluid volume	Chorioamnionitis, chorioamniotic membrane separation, PPROM, fetal urinary ascites, adjacent organ energy delivery
Serial amnioinfusion	Restore amniotic fluid volume, lower risk of PPROM than shunts or cystoscopy	Chorioamnionitis, chorioamniotic membrane separation, PPROM
Serial vesicocentesis	Unclear; normal amniotic fluid volume after bladder tap reported in some cases	Chorioamnionitis, chorioamniotic membrane separation, PPROM, fetal urinary ascites, abdominal wall defect, visceral injury
LUTO due to prolapsed ureterocele		
Needle puncture, laser ablation, balloon dilation	Potential for definitive treatment of the obstruction, restore amniotic fluid volume	Chorioamnionitis, chorioamniotic membrane separation, PPROM, fetal urinary ascites, failure to decompress in approximately 10%

Shunts have even been placed fetoscopically antegrade through the penis[11] instead of the traditional approach of entry through the abdominal wall. This requires a larger uterine opening, as it requires fetoscopic guidance, and it is not clear that instrumenting the fetal urethra so early in gestation results in reliably normal development; this should be considered experimental.

Fetal Cystoscopy

There were initially high hopes for fetal cystoscopy in the treatment of LUTO, and this is intuitive—if shunts dislodge and a postnatal surgery is necessary as the primary problem is untreated, averting both is ideal. The first case was performed in 1995 with fetal cystoscopy and valve fulguration[12] and a series reported the same year.[13] In this procedure, a fetoscope is placed either purely percutaneously or through the uterus after open exposure of the uterus and into the fetal bladder. The puncture through the fetal abdomen is higher toward the dome (shunt punctures are lower) to allow the best chance of bladder neck visualization. A curved fetoscope helps achieve this view.

A multicenter report on 40 fetal cystoscopies with 23 laser cases reported a survival rate of 60.9%. Unfortunately, four of the treated cases

(17%) had some form of urinary fistula. There were two cases of rectourethral fistula and two cases of urethra-cutaneous fistula, but the findings are more severe than the fistula alone—one case of urethrorectal fistula also was accompanied by atrophy of the gluteal muscle, and one case of urethrocutaneous fistula had a perineal tissue defect and limb atrophy (pregnancy was terminated). The likely reason for these failures is that the posterior urethra has a steep angle, around 70° in the prostatic urethra, and if energy is delivered more posteriorly a tissue injury may occur.[14]

Amnioinfusion

Infusion of amniotic fluid has been performed in two ways. The first is an amnioport, a technique principally used at Cincinnati Children's Hospital.[15] In these cases, a vascular access port is placed subcutaneously in the mother, and the uterus accessed by small laparotomy. A tunnel is created in the uterine wall to discourage leakage of amniotic fluid, and serial amnioinfusions performed. The port is then removed at delivery. There are cases of PPROM resulting in delivery with fatal pulmonary hypoplasia, but in most of the cases, the goal is accomplished and amniotic fluid is maintained for the remainder of the pregnancy. This technology has approached that has been used in cases of bilateral renal agenesis (BRA). In a series of two cases, one treated with an amnioport and the other with serial amnioinfusion, both survived to term; neither survived to transplantation.[16] Although it carries the advantage of requiring only a single (albeit invasive) access to the amniotic space, the approach has largely been supplanted by serial needle-delivered amnioinfusion.

The second technique is serial instillation of isotonic fluid through 20g or 22g ultrasound-guided needle placement into the amniotic space. This is commonly used for oligohydramnios due to preterm rupture of membranes (ie, a non-fetal source of low amniotic fluid)—published rates for chorioamnionitis and other complications are approximately 1/300 per infusion.[17] Based on this and the low survival rate for fetal BRA, the renal anhydramnios fetal therapy (RAFT) trial was initiated.[18,19] Inclusion criteria included anhydramnios before 22 weeks, and first amnioinfusion before 26 weeks with exclusions for abnormal karyotype or microarray, other associated abnormalities, or evidence of preterm labor. The goal of this ongoing trial is to plan to recruit 70 maternal/fetal pairs to undergo serial amnioinfusions. Warmed isotonic fluid, either normal saline or lactated ringers, will be instilled every 2 to 12 days with the frequency determined by the treating team. The primary outcome is postnatal survival of 15 continuous days. This is by far the largest prospective trial addressing LUTO ever conducted, and the results will provide the highest level of evidence regarding the effective of serial amnioinfusion. It should be noted that amnioinfusion, while seen to be associated with survival in several fetal cases, has substantial risks and is not clearly associated with prevention of pulmonary hypoplasia clinically or preclinically.[20]

Although the larger trial's data are not available to review at this time, we have important data to review for a portion of the subjects.[21] The RAFT trial recruited cases of oligo and anhydramnios from LUTO as well as a distinct group BRA; the BRA results were reported recently in the form an abstract in 2023. The results were profoundly sobering. Of the 20 dyads (mothers and fetuses) enrolled for BRA, there were 18 live births (90%), and 14 (70%) survived to 14 days after delivery with dialysis access placed. During pregnancy, chorioamniotic separation occurred in six cases. Although half of these separations occurred in the non-surviving fetuses, suggesting a worse prognosis, the difference between the arms was not significant. Nine (64%) experienced PPROM, occurring at a median of 66 days from the first amnioinfusion in the surviving arms and 22 days in those that did not survive (P = .013). As this is not a randomized trial, it is difficult to say if the membrane separation was causal with respect the poor survival or an effect of the condition. Accessing the amniotic space with absent fluid is technically challenging, and instillation of fluid resulting in iatrogenic membrane separation is possible. Preterm delivery was common; median gestational age was 33 weeks (IQR 32–3) for the survivors, and birthweight was 2010 gm (IQR 1840–2262.5). Complications were common and severe—seven surviving infants experienced stroke (50%), six experienced infections (43%), and there were two (14%) cases of necrotizing enterocolitis. The investigators summarize their outcomes with clarity and honesty: "5/14 infants who met the primary outcome survived to discharge on peritoneal dialysis (PD) at a median age of 25 w [IQR 12, 32]; 2 of the 5 died after discharge. 3 of the 5 infants discharged home and one who remains in the NICU sustained strokes." This is to say that of the 20 patients enrolled with BRA, no more than six survived to discharge with PD established, and all but two discharged babies had neurologic complications. The babies surviving to discharge did so after a median hospital stay of nearly half a year. After Data Safety Monitoring Board review, this arm of the study is suspended. The findings parallel that from retrospective cohorts of amnioinfusion for BRA.[16] The lessons from this reach beyond BRA, for which amnioinfusion will not again be performed, and speak to expectations of clinicians and families, and the special considerations that attend fetal interventions and trials.

Vesicocentesis

The role of aspirating urine from the fetal bladder alone, as a therapeutic intervention without any adjuvant procedure, is uncertain. There are cases in which the intervention is performed, and after two or more aspirations, the remainder of the pregnancy continues without a dilated bladder, with restoration of normal amniotic fluid volume, and without evident fistulous communication between the bladder and the amniotic space. To understand how peculiar this is, it is worth considering normal fetal renal physiology. The rate of fetal urinary production is surprisingly rapid, especially given fetal body weight.[22]

The standard noninvasive way to measure this is continuous ultrasound monitoring of the bladder, capturing 2D ultrasound images of the bladder in two planes, waiting for bladder filling and measuring this change in volume over time to calculate a rate. Fägerquist and colleagues found rates of 4 mL/h at 20 weeks, 12.1 mL/h at 25 weeks, 22.7 mL/h at 30 weeks, 36 mL/h at 35 weeks, and 52.2 mL/h at 40 weeks. For a World Health Organization median birthweight male baby of 7 lb 6 oz,[23] we can calculate that this corresponds to over 15 mL/kg/h. This is a great faster than urine production after birth[a]. In children, renal dysplasia often presents with polyuria and in LUTO anuric renal failure occurs, but is rare.[24] It is unclear to what degree urine production changes in LUTO. Even the most severe cases of LUTO, with over 100 cc of urine at 20 weeks, would be expected to refill within 24 hours at standard rates of fill. It is then unclear what the single bladder aspiration achieved physiologically.

Although we do not recommend vesicocentesis as a primary form of therapy, there are cases in which the intervention is performed, the imaging dramatically improves, and the diagnosis of PUV is confirmed postnatally.[25] It is possible these are the rare cases of spontaneous improvement of LUTO findings in utero, but it remains opaque and prediction of this is not possible.

Special Cases: Megalourethra

Fetoscopic treatment of megalourethra by meatotomy has been reported by a group in Mexico. The investigators report on 226 cases of LUTO, 10 with megalourethra, and three selected for intervention. The cohort construction here is critical; this represents a carefully selected cohort of an unusual cause of LUTO. These cases were treated around 21 weeks (as early as 18 weeks). Analogous to fetal shunting and fetal cystoscopy, amnioinfusion was performed and fetal paralysis administered. Through an 8Fr trocar, a 1.2-mm fetoscope with a curved sheal was used. They used a 400-nM diode laser to treat a thin membrane over the presumed orthotopic location of the urethral meatus, and the urethra gently inspected or probed. There was one fetal loss due to PPROM; the other survived to term with normal renal function after delivery.

Enthusiasm for this should be tempered not only by the case of fetal loss, but also by the existence of that cases of apparent fetal megalourethra resolve without any intervention at all.[26] This said, there is currently no way to predict which cases will resolve, and which cases may progress to experience umbilical cord compression or other complications from anhydramnios. We emphasize that the anatomy of the megalourethra does not normally permit this type of treatment—scaphoid megalourethras will have intact corpus spongiosum distally, precluding access with the fetoscope, and making any treatment hazardous and likely accompanies by bleeding. In most cases, observation is appropriate.

Special Cases: Ureterocele

Treatment of a prolapsing ureterocele resulting in LUTO has been reported. Although most ureteroceles do not impact the pregnancy at all, and treatment should be deferred until after delivery, it is true that a prolapsing ureterocele may result in fetal LUTO, and the results from intervention are favorable. Interestingly, there are several ways to address the ureterocele surgically, and none has been proven more effective than any other approach.[27,28] The most invasive option is fetoscopy—a 9Fr trocar is placed into the fetal bladder after paralytics. The ureterocele is incised with the Diode laser, and the ureterocele is further disrupted by moving the endoscope laterally to widen the laser-created aperture. An ultrasound-guided laser puncture is similar, but instead of using an endoscope a 20g needle is passed into the bladder. The laser fiber is inserted through this, and energy delivered by the diode laser. This has the advantage of creating a substantially smaller uterine opening but requires purely sonographic (instead of optical) guidance. Balloon puncture is performed by placing an 18g needle into the bladder, placing a balloon through this, dilating it to 3 mm, and the balloon withdrawn to rupture the ureterocele. The balloon is then in the bladder lumen, where it is deflated and withdrawn. We recommend proceeding with the least invasive option first, which are needle-based, ultrasound-guided intervention.

A principle of fetal surgery emphasized here is to achieve the anatomic intervention for the fetus with the smallest possibly uterine puncture. There is a tradeoff between greater precision of optically guided procedures and increase in risk. For example, fetoscopic tracheal balloon occlusion for congenital diaphragmatic hernia, intervention increases the odds of postnatal survival but also increases the odds of preterm labor and rupture of membranes.[29] Confusingly, needles are often expressed in Birmingham Wire Gauge,[30] which is medicine is commonly called gauge, although

---

[a]A useful rule of thumb for the reader is that approximately 4 cc/h is produced at the 20 weeks mid-gestation mark, and then urine production increases by 2 cc/h each subsequent week following. This is only approximate, and the investigators' regression above has a more accurate fit with a second-order polynomial. This said, with the exception of a fetus at term, this "back of the envelope" approximation the authors use fits within one standard deviation of the true value; the authors have not encountered a clinical situation in which more precision was required.

multiple wire gauge scales exist in engineering. Charrière's eponymous scale (hence the older term Ch), now called a French Scale (Fr) after his nationality, is used for catheters, and some interventional sheaths are simply the diameter in millimeters times three. These are often used side by side; a conversion of commonly seen gauges in fetal surgery to diameters (mm) and French (Fr) is provided (**Table 2**). Note that a fetoscope is 1.2 mm in diameter (3.6Fr), and a 15g needle (approximately 5.4Fr) has an internal diameter of 1.37 mm; below this diameter, no optically guided interventions are possible.

RENAL OUTCOMES FROM RELIEF OF OBSTRUCTION

It is rational to assume that intervention to relieve urologic obstruction may avert some of the CKD known to result in cases of LUTO. It is similarly tempting to believe that perhaps the remarkable healing known to occur in fetal conditions could perhaps reverse renal dysplasia. At present, there are no convincing data that the relief of urologic obstruction improves renal outcomes postnatally.

Hope for this arose again this year in a manuscript from Germany, using the Somatex shunt and concluding that early intervention before 16 weeks may result in improved pulmonary and renal outcomes.[31] The investigators report on a series of 63 consecutive cases receiving a shunt. Intriguingly, they note that of the surviving fetuses with follow-up and treated early, before 17 weeks, versus those

treated after this, 15/19 had normal renal function, whereas only 9/28 fetuses treated later did. Although this may seem to compel early treatment, an accompanying paper nicely displays the concerns. We share Dr Farrugia's caution regarding this article in that in the study above in that postnatal diagnosis is heterogenous or unknown in one-third of the cohort (ie, not clear that PUV was causing obstruction) that renal outcome is defined only at hospital discharge and no further, and many of the treated babies had ultrasonographically abnormal kidneys.[32] As a cautionary side note, even with high-volume centers publishing top outcomes with improved shunts, 14% of the cohort experienced fetal demise after the intervention.

FETAL URINARY ASCITES

Any puncture of the bladder may result in ascites. This seems to be quite common, even following relatively benign interventions such as vesicocentesis.[33] The true rate is not known. A recent study from a large center reviewed their experience with shunt placement for urinary ascites—of the 10 cases of fetal LUTO for whom a peritoneo-amniotic shunt was placed, six were for ascites after bladder tap, three were for shunt dislodgement, and only one for spontaneous bladder perforation. The results were relatively favorable compared with shunts for LUTO, with two cases of shunt failure, presumed to be due to obstruction from bowel, and only one case of ventral hernia from an abdominal wall defect.[34] The natural history of iatrogenic urinary ascites is not clear.

ETHICS

The above has addressed "how" of fetal intervention, but the more difficult questions both clinically and for research are "should." A full discussion of the ethics of intervention is beyond the scope of this article, but there are specific reasons to pause and focus on this here. Intervention for BRA received intense press coverage in 2014 after amnioinfusion was performed in a case of anhydramnios and the baby was born. The long-term outcome for the specific pregnancy was not known either at the time of CNN's reporting or in the literature,[20] but the news reports impacting the hopes and clinical considerations for other pregnancies. The headfirst inclination to intervene, especially when positive clinical outcomes are shown, must be weighed against caution regarding full knowledge of the clinical condition, gaps in the causal certainty regarding diagnosis, and outcome, and Dr Harrison's admonition to consider risk.

Table 2 Common instrument outer diameters in fetal intervention			
	Gauge	Millimeters[a]	French
Amniocentesis needle (general use, paralytic injection)	22	0.7	2.1
Amniocentesis needle (general use)	20	0.9	2.7
Introduction of balloon angiocatheter	18	1.3	3.9
Harrison shunt system	15	1.8	5.4
Rocket shunt system (approximate)	10	3.3	9.9

[a] Nominal outer diameter.

PSYCHOSOCIAL CONSIDERATIONS

The impact of a LUTO diagnosis on the family is tremendous. Wide extrapolations across national borders and specific diagnoses should be discouraged, but we find the interviews conducted with the 10 Swedish women to be reveal important themes that we frequently encounter in our practice.[35] This is the only qualitative research available studying exclusively the impact of fetal urologic diagnoses on expectant mothers. The women describe four categories of feelings:

1. "Being prepared," now that an unexpected finding has been discovered.
2. "Living in suspense during pregnancy." The anxiety associated with this is substantial.
3. "Suppress feelings and hope for the best." Anyone who has participated in prenatal counseling will occasionally see overt manifestations of this, a form of compartmentalizing the uncomfortable feeling that accompanies this diagnosis.
4. "Difficulty in understanding information." The women had the impression that they had incomplete knowledge of the medical condition. We think there are three important, and actionable, points here.
   a. The first is that there may be true diagnostic uncertainty, in which case being frank with the family regarding medicine's limits, as distinct from any limits in the family's comprehension, are the primary factor.
   b. Second, to understand that in the setting of a severe diagnosis, it is difficult to absorb information. This is true both intuitively and scientifically; there is copious evidence that it is common that patient's understanding is incomplete when a serious diagnosis is given and potential toxic therapeutics are being considered. At a major teaching hospital, of 125 patients undergoing chemotherapy for a newly diagnosed solid malignancy, the goals of care were concordant in only 25% of cases.[36] Non-native English speakers had nearly 80% lower odds of concordance, but printed material given during the consent process increased concordance nearly threefold. In other studies, concordance between patient and provider plans for chemotherapy is low as 25%; the need for monitoring for what a family has internalized versus what has been communicated is paramount.[37]
   c. Last, to understand this point exactly as the investigators communicated—the women felt that they did not have complete

understanding. They actually may have absorbed precisely the understanding of the practitioners hope to convey, but the feeling of incomplete comprehension is legitimate, uncomfortable, and common. Some feelings, and the resulting actions, that prenatal testing produces may be surprising.[38] In a large study of over 80 reports on prenatal diagnosis, "providing or receiving ultrasound was positive for most, reportedly increasing parental-fetal engagement. However, abnormal findings were often shocking. Some reported changing future reproductive decisions after equivocal results, even when the eventual diagnosis was positive." The idea that favorable news would result in negative feelings or caution regarding future diagnoses should be on the minds of the clinicians.

To reiterate the importance of mental health in prenatal diagnosis, a large prospective study was performed using the Perinatal Anxiety Screening Scale.[39] The investigators found the highest anxiety was highest in second/third trimesters: subjects aged age 24 or younger, those with a history of anxiety, or with prior pregnancy loss. After the ultrasound, anxiety scores decreased except for those whose ultrasound results were indeterminate, again underscoring the importance of the feelings of uncertainty.

SUMMARY

There have been significant advancements in sonographic quality, MRI, shunt materials, endoscopic optics, endoscopic light delivery, laser application, clinical research quality, and the diffusion of medical knowledge since 1982. Despite this, fetal intervention on the urinary tract remains hazardous, and prenatally the authors remain often unable to provide the secure diagnoses which families' desire. The authors advocate approaching prenatal intervention with humility, understanding the data, the limitations, and the psychosocial needs of families receiving a LUTO diagnosis who deserve our empathy and compassion.

REFERENCES

1. Liley AW. Intrauterine transfusion of foetus in haemolytic disease. Br Med J 1963;2(5365):1107–9.
2. Harrison MR, Golbus MS, Filly RA, et al. Fetal surgery for congenital hydronephrosis. N Engl J Med 1982;306(10):591–3.
3. Ruano R, Sananes N, Wilson C, et al. Fetal lower urinary tract obstruction: proposal for standardized

multidisciplinary prenatal management based on disease severity. Ultrasound Obstet Gynecol 2016; 48(4):476–82.

4. Ruano R, Dunn T, Braun MC, et al. Lower urinary tract obstruction: fetal intervention based on prenatal staging. Pediatr Nephrol 2017;32(10):1871–8.

5. Fontanella F, Groen H, Duin LK, et al. Z-scores of fetal bladder size for antenatal differential diagnosis between posterior urethral valves and urethral atresia. Ultrasound Obstet Gynecol 2021;58(6): 875–81.

6. Kurtz MP, Koh CJ, Jamail GA, et al. Factors associated with fetal shunt dislodgement in lower urinary tract obstruction. Prenat Diagn 2016;36(8):720–5.

7. Morris RK, Malin GL, Quinlan-Jones E, et al. Percutaneous vesicoamniotic shunting versus conservative management for fetal lower urinary tract obstruction (PLUTO): a randomised trial. Lancet 2013;382(9903):1496–506.

8. Morris RK, Malin GL, Quinlan-Jones E, et al. The Percutaneous shunting in Lower Urinary Tract Obstruction (PLUTO) study and randomised controlled trial: evaluation of the effectiveness, cost-effectiveness and acceptability of percutaneous vesicoamniotic shunting for lower urinary tract obstruction. Health Technol Assess 2013;17(59): 1–232.

9. Strizek B, Spicher T, Gottschalk I, et al. Vesicoamniotic Shunting before 17 + 0 Weeks in Fetuses with Lower Urinary Tract Obstruction (LUTO): Comparison of Somatex vs. Harrison Shunt Systems. J Clin Med 2022;11(9). https://doi.org/10.3390/jcm11092359.

10. Keil C, Bedei I, Sommer L, et al. Fetal therapy of LUTO (lower urinary tract obstruction) - a follow-up observational study. J Matern Fetal Neonatal Med 2022;35(25):8536–43.

11. Hofmann R, Becker T, Meyer-Wittkopf M, et al. Fetoscopic placement of a transurethral stent for intrauterine obstructive uropathy. J Urol 2004;171(1): 384–6.

12. Quintero RA, Hume R, Msith C, et al. Percutaneous fetal cystoscopy and endoscopic fulguration of posterior urethral valves. Am J Obstet Gynecol 1995; 172(1):206–9.

13. Quintero RA, Johnson MP, Romero R, et al. In-utero percutaneous cystoscopy in the management of fetal lower obstructive uropathy. Lancet 1995; 346(8974):537–40.

14. Sananes N, Favre R, Koh CJ, et al. Urological fistulas after fetal cystoscopic laser ablation of posterior urethral valves: surgical technical aspects. Ultrasound Obstet Gynecol 2015;45(2): 183–9.

15. Polzin WJ, Lim FY, Habli M, et al. Use of an Amnioport to Maintain Amniotic Fluid Volume in Fetuses with Oligohydramnios Secondary to Lower Urinary Tract Obstruction or Fetal Renal Anomalies. Fetal Diagn Ther 2017;41(1):51–7.

16. Riddle S, Habli M, Tabbah S, et al. Contemporary Outcomes of Patients with Isolated Bilateral Renal Agenesis with and without Fetal Intervention. Fetal Diagn Ther 2020;47(9):675–81.

17. Werner EF, Hauspurg A, Bienstock JL. In-utero treatment of bilateral renal agenesis: a threshold analysis of possible cost effectiveness. Obstet Gynecol Int J 2015;2(3).

18. O'hare EM, Jelin AC, Miller JL, et al. Amnioinfusions to Treat Early Onset Anhydramnios Caused by Renal Anomalies: Background and Rationale for the Renal Anhydramnios Fetal Therapy Trial. Fetal Diagn Ther 2019;45(6):365–72.

19. Jelin AC, Sagaser KG, Forster KR, et al. Etiology and management of early pregnancy renal anhydramnios: Is there a place for serial amnioinfusions? Prenat Diagn 2020;40(5):528–37.

20. Johnson A, Luks FI. A cautionary note on new fetal interventions. Obstet Gynecol 2014;124(2 Pt 2 Suppl 1):411–2.

21. Miller JL, Baschat AA, Rosner M, et al. Neonatal survival after serial amnioinfusions for fetal bilateral renal agenesis: report from the raft trial. Am J Obstet Gynecol 2023;228(1):S766–7.

22. Fägerquist M, Fägerquist U, Odén A, et al. Fetal urine production and accuracy when estimating fetal urinary bladder volume. Ultrasound Obstet Gynecol 2001;17(2):132–9.

23. World Health Organization Standards for Age. Available at: https://www.who.int/tools/child-growth-standards/standards/weight-for-age. Accessed February 1, 2023.

24. Ruano R, Safdar A, Au J, et al. Defining and predicting 'intrauterine fetal renal failure' in congenital lower urinary tract obstruction. Pediatr Nephrol 2016; 31(4):605–12.

25. Pahlitzsch T, Dressler I, Henrich W, et al. EP24.01: Serial vesicocentesis as successful treatment of LUTO. Ultrasound Obstet Gynecol 2019;54(S1): 391–2.

26. Nijagal A, Sydorak RM, Feldstein VA, et al. Spontaneous resolution of prenatal megalourethra. J Pediatr Surg 2004;39(9):1421–3.

27. Sepúlveda-González G, Villagomez-Martínez GE, Arroyo-Lemarroy T, et al. Fetal surgery for obstructive ureterocele using an ultrasound-guided needle laser ablation technique: a case series. J Matern Fetal Neonatal Med 2022;35(25). https://doi.org/10.1080/14767058.2022.2061345.

28. Chalouhi GE, Morency AM, de Vlieger R, et al. Prenatal incision of ureterocele causing bladder outlet obstruction: a multicenter case series. Prenat Diagn 2017;37(10):968–74.

29. Deprest JA, Nicolaides KH, Benachi A, et al. Randomized Trial of Fetal Surgery for Severe Left

Diaphragmatic Hernia. N Engl J Med 2021;385(2): 107–18.

30. "Sigma Aldrich." Syringe Needle Conversion Chart. Sigma Aldrich. Published 2023. Available at: https://www.sigmaaldrich.com/. Accessed February 1, 2023.

31. Kohl T, Fimmers R, Axt-Fliedner R, et al. Vesico-amniotic shunt insertion prior to the completion of 16 weeks results in improved preservation of renal function in surviving fetuses with isolated severe lower urinary tract obstruction (LUTO). J Pediatr Urol 2022;18(2):116–26.

32. Farrugia MK. Vesico-amniotic shunt insertion prior to the completion of 16 weeks results in improved preservation of renal function in surviving fetuses with isolated severe lower urinary tract obstruction (LUTO). J Pediatr Urol 2022;18(2):129–30.

33. Hidaka N, Chiba Y. Transient Urinary Ascites after Vesicocentesis Observed in a Fetus with Megacystis Caused by Posterior Urethral Valve. Fetal Diagn Ther 2009;25(2):192–5.

34. Donepudi R, Shamshirsaz AA, Espinoza J, et al. Peritoneal-amniotic shunt in management of urinary ascites complicating fetal lower urinary tract obstruction. Ultrasound Obstet Gynecol 2021; 58(2):320–2.

35. Oscarsson M, Gottvall T, Swahnberg K. When fetal hydronephrosis is suspected antenatally–a qualitative study. BMC Pregnancy Childbirth 2015;15:349. https://doi.org/10.1186/s12884-015-0791-x.

36. Lennes IT, Temel JS, Hoedt C, et al. Predictors of newly diagnosed cancer patients' understanding of the goals of their care at initiation of chemotherapy. Cancer 2013;119(3):691–9.

37. Almalki H, Absi A, Alghamdi A, et al. Analysis of Patient-Physician Concordance in the Understanding of Chemotherapy Treatment Plans Among Patients With Cancer. JAMA Netw Open 2020;3(3):e200341.

38. Moncrieff G, Finlayson K, Cordey S, et al. First and second trimester ultrasound in pregnancy: A systematic review and metasynthesis of the views and experiences of pregnant women, partners, and health workers. PLoS One 2021;16(12): e0261096.

39. Gross MS, Ju H, Osborne LM, et al. Indeterminate Prenatal Ultrasounds and Maternal Anxiety: A Prospective Cohort Study. Matern Child Health J 2021; 25(5):802–12.

Ureteropelvic Junction Obstruction/ Hydronephrosis

Peter Y. Cai, MD[a], Richard S. Lee, MD[a,b],*

KEYWORDS

- Hydronephrosis • Ureteropelvic junction obstruction • Pyeloplasty • Robotic surgery

KEY POINTS

- Congenital hydronephrosis is a common finding in the pediatric population that can commonly be managed conservatively.
- Additional work-up with diuretic renogram should be performed for patients with significant hydronephrosis in the absence of hydroureter to evaluate for ureteropelvic junction obstruction.
- Indications for surgical repair of ureteropelvic junction obstruction include recurrent pain crises, differential renal function less than 40%, decline in renal function over time, urinary tract infections, worsening hydronephrosis, or nephrolithiasis.
- Anderson-Hynes dismembered pyeloplasty repair has high success rates and uncommon complications regardless of surgical approach.

DIAGNOSIS OF CONGENITAL HYDRONEPHROSIS

Hydronephrosis, defined by dilatation of the collecting system in the upper urinary tract (ie, ureter, renal pelvis, major calyces, minor calyces), is a common urologic finding present in up to 2.3% of all pregnancies screened with fetal ultrasonography.[1–3] As a result, it is a common reason for pediatric urology referral either prenatally or during early infancy. When detected by prenatal screening ultrasound, this anomaly is referred to as antenatal hydronephrosis (ANH) and can have a wide range of differential diagnoses including vesicoureteral reflux or obstructive processes, such as urethral atresia, posterior urethral valve, ureterocele, megaureter, or ureteropelvic junction obstruction (UPJO). This article focuses on the diagnosis and management of UPJO; subsequent articles in this issue discuss the other congenital anomalies.

Patients with UPJO have obstruction resulting from narrowing of the junction between the renal pelvis and proximal ureter (**Fig. 1**). Without the technology to screen for ANH, UPJO historically presented with clinical signs and symptoms that required medical and surgical management. Today, ultrasound is part of routine prenatal care with significant improvements in morphologic assessment from modern technology and increasing utilization for obstetric patients.[4–6] With better detection of fetal abnormalities,[7] including ANH, it has become increasingly important to recognize the spectrum of severity to determine which cases can be managed conservatively. The current challenge is to use the abundance of information from routine prenatal screening to dictate proper patient management and counseling with a pediatric urologist.

In the absence of a classification system, early attempts at characterizing the spectrum of ANH used subjective terms, such as mild, moderate,

Funding: P.Y. Cai is supported by NIH, United States training grant (Award #T32DK060442–19).
[a] Department of Urology, Boston Children's Hospital, 300 Longwood Avenue, Hunnewell 390, Boston, MA 02115, USA; [b] Department of Surgery, Harvard Medical School, Boston Children's Hospital, 300 Longwood Avenue, Boston, MA 02115, USA
* Corresponding author.
E-mail address: richard.lee@childrens.harvard.edu

Urol Clin N Am 50 (2023) 361–369
https://doi.org/10.1016/j.ucl.2023.04.001

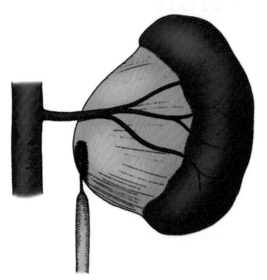

Fig. 1. Hydronephrosis secondary to intrinsic obstruction from narrowing of the junction between the renal pelvis and ureter. (*From* Campbell-Walsh-Wein 12th Edition, Chapter 42.)

and severe. In 1986, a morphologic classification system was proposed that included the antero-posterior renal pelvic diameter (APRPD) with cut-offs of less than 10 mm, 10 to 15 mm, or greater than 15 mm.[8] Subsequently, pediatric urologists from the Society for Fetal Urology (SFU) created the SFU grading system expecting that a numeric scale may be easier to learn and improve consistency across providers (**Table 1**).[9] However, this system has had major limitations including lack of data on correlation with risk and questionable interrater agreement.[10] Across different specialties, there was also significant variation in preference with obstetricians preferring the APRPD, whereas pediatric urologists and radiologists were split between APRPD and SFU grading.[11]

To address this variability, a consensus conference was held in 2014 among various specialties (obstetrics, radiology, urology, nephrology) to create a unified classification system that is now known as the Urinary Tract Dilation (UTD) classification system. This system establishes risk stratification in the prenatal and postnatal setting based on important imaging abnormalities, such as peripheral calyceal dilation, kidney parenchymal thickness and appearance, and ureteral and bladder abnormalities.[12] Despite the limitations in creating a comprehensive classification system, the degree of hydronephrosis is known to be a strong predictor of postnatal pathology (mild ANH associated with 11.9% and severe ANH associated with 88.3% risk of postnatal pathology).[13] Although not without controversy, the UTD system does incorporate imaging and clinical features to improve the ability to discriminate between those at high- and low-risk, is easy-to-learn, and has improved consistency among different providers across different practice settings (ie, interrater reliability).[14,15]

URINARY TRACT DILATION CLASSIFICATION SYSTEM

When using the UTD system, ANH is defined as either greater than 4 mm APRPD on second-trimester prenatal ultrasound (16–27 weeks) or greater than 7 mm APRPD on third-trimester ultrasound (≥28 weeks) (**Fig. 2**). Patients are classified as UTD A1 or low risk in the absence of large amounts of renal dilation (<7 mm in second trimester or <10 mm in third trimester) or other concerning features (peripheral calyceal dilation, renal parenchymal abnormalities, ureteral dilation, bladder abnormalities, and oligohydramnios). The presence of any of these findings defines the UTD A2–3 or increased risk categorization. The initial schema defined intermediate-risk (A2) and high-risk (A3) groups separately based on the presence of peripheral calyceal dilation, but was later combined after acknowledging the difficulty in distinguishing peripheral calyceal dilation on prenatal ultrasound.

Postnatal evaluation is stratified into three categories: low- (UTD P1), intermediate- (UTD P2), and high-risk (UTD P3) (**Fig. 3**). UTD P1 is defined as APRPD between 10 and 15 mm and absence of any other concerning imaging features. UTD P2 is defined as APRPD greater than or equal to 15 mm or presence of either peripheral calyceal dilation or ureteral dilation. Patients who have APRPD less than 15 mm but have peripheral calyceal dilation or ureteral dilation would still be classified as UTD P2 because these are considered risk-defining features. There cannot be any parenchymal (ie, thinning, increased echogenicity, decreased corticomedullary differentiation) or bladder abnormalities (ie, ureterocele, thickening), because these would define the high-risk UTD P3 category. Similarly, presence of any of these features with APRPD less than 15 mm would still be classified as UTD P3.

WORK-UP OF CONGENITAL HYDRONEPHROSIS

Fetal intervention for hydronephrosis is rarely indicated. Prenatal management of ANH typically focuses on determining frequency of prenatal ultrasounds, referral for consultations, and postnatal evaluation. For the low-risk UTD A1 cohort,

Table 1
Society for Fetal Urology grading system for antenatal hydronephrosis

Grade 0	No hydronephrosis
Grade 1	Only renal pelvis is dilated
Grade 2	Hydronephrosis is present in a few calyces
Grade 3	Virtually all calyces are dilated
Grade 4	Parenchymal thinning

an additional ultrasound is recommended after 32 weeks to evaluate for resolution of ANH and obviate postnatal follow-up (**Fig. 4**). For the increased-risk UTD A2–3 cohort, a follow-up prenatal ultrasound is recommended within 4 to 6 weeks of the diagnosis and subsequent studies are up to the discretion of the clinician based on the individual diagnoses; however, a voiding cystourethrogram (VCUG) is typically indicated. It is recommended for these patients to obtain prenatal consultation with a pediatric urologist and/or pediatric nephrologist because of increased risk for significant pathology or renal dysfunction. Both cohorts are recommended for postnatal ultrasound evaluation greater than 48 hours of life (unless posterior urethral valves or significant

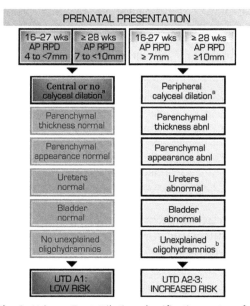

PRENATAL PRESENTATION

| 16–27 wks AP RPD 4 to <7mm | ≥ 28 wks AP RPD 7 to <10mm | 16-27 wks AP RPD ≥7mm | ≥ 28 wks AP RPD ≥10mm |

Central or no calyceal dilation[a] → Peripheral calyceal dilation[a]

Parenchymal thickness normal — Parenchymal thickness abnl

Parenchymal appearance normal — Parenchymal appearance abnl

Ureters normal — Ureters abnormal

Bladder normal — Bladder abnormal

No unexplained oligohydramnios — Unexplained oligohydramnios[b]

UTD A1: LOW RISK — UTD A2-3: INCREASED RISK

Fig. 2. Urinary Tract Dilation classification system for prenatal presentation. GU, genitourinary. [a]Central and peripheral calyceal dilation may be difficult to evaluate early in gestation. [b]Oligohydramnios is suspected to result from a GU cause. (*From* Nguyen H, et al. J Pediatr Urol 2014.)

bladder outlet obstruction are suspected) because earlier imaging is associated with false-negative results from a combination of relative state of dehydration and low glomerular filtration rate in neonates.[16]

After obtaining postnatal ultrasound, patients are again risk-categorized as discussed in the prior section to determine further management. Follow-up ultrasound is recommended in 1 to 6 months for UTD P1, 1 to 3 months for UTD P2, and 1 month for UTD P3 (**Fig. 5**). Although additional work-up with functional scan, VCUG, and prophylactic antibiotics are left to the discretion of the clinician based on the pathology suspected, patients with UTD P3 are recommended to undergo a VCUG and be considered for prophylactic antibiotics. These topics are discussed in more detail in a subsequent section on vesicoureteral reflux.

A significant proportion of postnatal hydronephrosis (41%) self-resolves over time. This natural history varies by UTD risk score ($P < .001$), with lower amounts of resolution in patients with higher risk scores.[17] In addition, UTD P3 patients are at higher risk for needing surgical intervention on follow-up, with 46% of P3 undergoing surgery versus 1% of P0, 1% of P1, and 6% of P2 ($P < .001$). These data support the utility of this scoring system in identifying the highest risk patients in clinical practice and counseling families. However, there is controversy regarding the appropriate management for low-risk patients because patients with UTD P1 had no difference in outcomes compared with patients without hydronephrosis, yet repeat ultrasounds are still performed and require significant resource utilization.[18]

Patients with significant hydronephrosis in the absence of hydroureter and vesicoureteral reflux should be worked up for UPJO with a diuretic renogram scan, such as a technetium-99m mercaptoacetyltriglycine-3 (MAG3), to determine relative differential renal function and evaluate for functional obstruction. Briefly, this imaging study involves injection of a radiotracer that is secreted by the proximal tubules to estimate renal function and also uses intravenous diuretic (ie, furosemide) to facilitate radiotracer excretion from the collecting system. Drainage from the collecting system is measured using the time from furosemide injection until 50% of maximum radiotracer value remains (T ½), with greater than 20 minutes conventionally used as a cutoff for significant obstruction.[19] However, this value should not be used alone to rule out obstruction because the study can be inaccurate with poor renal function; in the presence of a massively dilated collecting

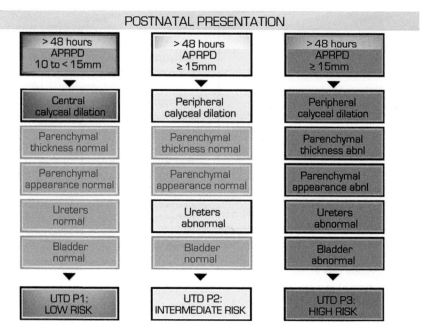

Fig. 3. Urinary Tract Dilation classification system for postnatal presentation. (*From* Nguyen H, et al. J Pediatr Urol 2014.)

system; and with complex anatomy, such as concomitant ureterovesical junction obstruction. Although there are published guidelines on the role of intravenous hydration, urethral catheterization, and administration of diuretics, these practices are not consistent across all centers.[20]

MRI urography has also been studied as an alternative to conventional ultrasound and MAG3 renal scans and was found to be comparable in functional assessment of obstruction with superior anatomic detail and eliminates the need for neonatal radiation exposure.[21] Despite these advantages, the need for sedation, availability, and costs have limited its widespread adoption.

More recently, biomarkers have been extensively studied as an alternative to assessing renal parenchymal status.[22] For example, urine samples from patients undergoing pyeloplasty were found to have levels of extracellular matrix proteins and enzymes that predict reduced renal function on MAG3 scan.[23] Although additional studies are necessary before biomarkers are practical in the clinical setting, they offer the invaluable potential for a noninvasive method to identify which patients are at highest risk for deterioration and surgical intervention.

Historically, hydronephrosis secondary to UPJO was primarily treated with timely surgical correction (ie, pyeloplasty) to prevent additional renal parenchymal changes and maximize lifelong renal function.[24] However, long-term follow-up after

nonoperative management showed that approximately 80% of cases completely resolved or had improved hydronephrosis.[25,26] These and other studies that examined clinical findings, radiographic imaging, and renal biopsies all suggest that UPJO is a congenital disorder with a wide spectrum that ranges from self-resolving in a large majority to necessitating surgical repair in a minority of patients.[27] Indications for surgical repair are still controversial but include recurrent pain crises, differential renal function less than 40%, decline in renal function over time, urinary tract infections, worsening hydronephrosis, or nephrolithiasis. In the absence of these concerning features, management begins with surveillance using serial ultrasounds and diuretic renogram scans given the high likelihood of self-resolution and successful management with a conservative approach.

SURGICAL MANAGEMENT OF URETEROPELVIC JUNCTION OBSTRUCTION
Preoperative Planning

In patients undergoing pyeloplasty, preoperative planning involves obtaining the appropriate imaging studies and determining which surgical approach is most suitable for the patient. Preoperative laboratory testing can include urine culture and serum tests for kidney function.

In most children with UPJO identified after a prenatal or early postnatal evaluation, a VCUG has

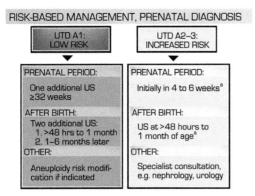

Fig. 4. Management recommendations based on Urinary Tract Dilation classification system for prenatal presentation. US, ultrasound. [a]Certain situations (eg, posterior urethral valves, bilateral severe hydronephrosis) may require more expedient follow up. (*From* Nguyen H, et al. J Pediatr Urol 2014.)

Pyeloplasty is the gold standard for repair. Pyeloplasty is performed in many different approaches, including open retroperitoneal, dorsal lumbotomy, laparoscopic transperitoneal or retroperitoneal, and robotic transperitoneal or retroperitoneal. The original description of the surgical management of UPJO by Anderson and Hynes in 1949 was an open approach, followed by the first report of laparoscopic pyeloplasty in 1995, and the introduction of the pediatric robotic-assisted laparoscopic pyeloplasty (RALP) in the 2000s.[32,33] Open repair through a flank incision or anterior abdominal approach allows for an extraperitoneal approach. These approaches typically provide excellent exposure and visualization of the anatomy. The posterior/dorsal lumbotomy incision, which has the oldest historical origin with the first report by Simon in 1870 and repopularization in the pediatric population by several groups in the 1980s,[34–36] is another open approach. Although the dorsal lumbotomy offers the most direct path to the ureteropelvic junction and a small incision, there are limitations in exposure, particularly in older children. Additionally, identification of crossing vessels is difficult in the dorsal lumbotomy approach.

Laparoscopic repair is associated with shorter hospital stays and decreased narcotic use in older children with no differences in outcomes.[37] Despite these benefits, the technical challenges and steep learning curve of conventional laparoscopic suturing may have contributed to its lack of popularity. The introduction of robotic technology has answered this challenge by providing improved visualization and magnification, finer instruments with greater degrees of freedom, and enhanced dexterity. As a result, RALP has been rapidly adopted and accounted for 40% of pyeloplasty repairs in the United States in 2015.[38,39] Although there has been concern about the

been performed for the evaluation of UTD P2 or P3. In children or adolescents identified with UPJO later in life, VCUG is typically not performed unless there is a history of febrile urinary tract infection or ureteral dilation. It is also important to consider that UPJO can be caused by intrinsic narrowing (see **Fig. 1**) or extrinsic obstruction from a crossing vessel (**Fig. 6**). Age of presentation and history typically point toward a specific cause. Patients who present at younger age with ANH most commonly have intrinsic narrowing, whereas older children and adults who present with symptoms have approximately 50% risk of extrinsic obstruction from a crossing vessel.[28,29] Although some have advocated for MRI and color Doppler imaging to rule out crossing vessels, its value is questionable because surgical correction is required and ultimately is dictated by intraoperative findings.[30,31]

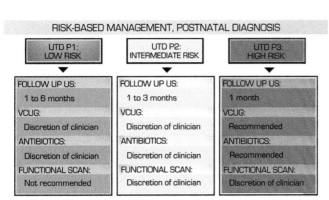

The choice to utilize prophylactic antibiotics or recommend voiding cystourethrogram will depend on the suspected underlying pathology

Fig. 5. Management recommendations based on Urinary Tract Dilation classification system for postnatal presentation. (*From* Nguyen H, et al. J Pediatr Urol 2014.)

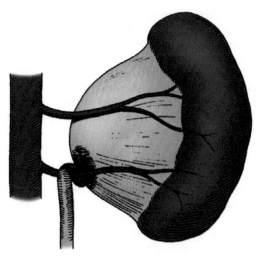

Fig. 6. Hydronephrosis secondary to extrinsic obstruction from crossing vessel. (*From* Campbell-Walsh-Wein 12th Edition, Chapter 42.)

robotic approach in young infants because of limited operative space and the risk associated with increased operative time, single-institution and multicenter studies have demonstrated that RALP is safely performed in infants less than 10 kg or less than 1 year of age.[40,41] The following sections specifically discuss the robotic transperitoneal approach with Anderson-Hynes dismembered pyeloplasty, although we acknowledge that there is still an important role for other approaches. Endopyelotomy is uncommonly used in children. It is associated with lower success and higher complication rates compared with the gold standard pyeloplasty repair.[42]

Preparation and Positioning

Our department's standard protocol incorporates elements of Enhanced Recovery After Surgery including minimally invasive approach when possible, nausea prophylaxis, and minimizing pain control.[43] Preoperatively, we encourage hydration with oral carbohydrate liquid (ie, Pedialyte or Gatorade) to maintain euvolemia and minimize risk for postoperative kidney injury. For older children, we encourage them to have a bowel movement before surgery but no longer prescribe laxatives. Younger infants are asked to follow standard preoperative anesthesia oral intake guidelines. Although some favor starting with retrograde pyelography because of the reported possibility of distal obstruction and narrowing or ureteral polyp, we have found that this is unnecessary in the presence of high-quality preoperative imaging studies and in the absence of hydroureter.[44,45] However, if preoperative imaging is

unclear or if reoperative surgery is being performed, retrograde pyelography is a valuable tool to better define the ureteral anatomy.

Prophylactic antibiotics should be administered as recommended for clean-contaminated case in the genitourinary tract and broadened for patients with multidrug-resistant organisms on preoperative urine culture. Before positioning, a Foley catheter is placed for bladder drainage and to allow for retrograde fluid instillation in later steps to confirm appropriate anterograde stent placement. We routinely send the bladder urine for culture at the time of catheter placement to determine if postoperative antibiotics are needed. The patient is then placed in the modified lateral decubitus position with the ipsilateral side supported by wedge or gel roll. The contralateral arm is flexed and placed on a padded arm board, and the ipsilateral arm is placed on the side of the patient in anatomic position. A combination of foam padding, towels, and tape is used to secure the patient while taking care to protect the skin and pad any pressure points. Extra time is spent on ensuring the neck is in normal anatomic position and padded to prevent traction or pressure injury. The catheter tubing should be easily accessible to the circulating nurse or bedside assistant after subsequent positioning. In males, the Foley catheter is often placed on the field after positioning and draping for easier access.

Surgical Steps

- Open Hasson technique to gain access to the peritoneal cavity and place the initial periumbilical 8-mm camera port (da Vinci Xi system) under vision with a 5-mm 0° laparoscopic lens.
- Pneumoperitoneum is set to 12 mm Hg and additional ports are placed under direct vision.
- Two additional ports are placed taking care to maximize working space and minimize collisions: one cranial to the camera port in midline, and one caudal either toward the anterior superior iliac spine or at midline depending on available space. Hidden incision endoscopic surgery technique for port placement can also be used when appropriate.[46]
- An additional 5-mm assistant port can be placed to facilitate exposure (liver or spleen) but is extremely uncommon outside of reoperative surgery.
- Once all ports are placed the pressure is dropped to 8 to 10 mm Hg. The remainder of the surgery is completed using a 30° camera lens.

- Procedure begins with exposing the renal pelvis with bipolar forceps in the left hand and monopolar scissors in the right hand. Left-sided cases can be approached transmesenteric. Otherwise, the colon is mobilized along the white line of Toldt to expose the retroperitoneal space.
- The gonadal vessels and proximal ureter are first identified. As the ureter is separated from the gonadal vessels, the ureter is mobilized proximally toward the renal pelvis. Posterior dissection toward the renal pelvis allows for safe detection of crossing vessels. Limited use of cautery is important to preserve blood supply to the ureter. After posterior dissection, the renal pelvis is freed anteriorly and superior to the UPJO. It is critical, particularly with crossing vessels, to minimize dissection and handling of the crossing vessels. The key concept is to mobilize the ureter and renal pelvis away from the crossing vessels.
- To assist with exposure, a hitch-stitch is placed percutaneously using 2–0 monofilament suture. The suture is passed through the renal pelvis just cranial and anteromedial to anticipated location of pyelotomy.
- Pyelotomy is performed using scissors without cautery proximal to the obstructed segment.
- The divided ureter is spatulated posterior laterally. Ureter is not resected until the end of the anastomosis to allow for easier manipulation of the ureter during the anastomosis.
- Posterior wall of anastomosis is completed first using either running or interrupted 6–0 monofilament suture.
- Before completion of the anterior anastomosis, a double-J ureteral stent is placed anterograde. A 14-gauge angiocatheter is placed percutaneously to allow for a straight approach to the anastomosis. An angled guidewire is passed through the angiocatheter and advanced into the anastomosis and down the ureter using hand-over-hand robotic technique. The double-J stent is advanced over the wire in a similar fashion and should easily pass into the bladder. Stent placement is confirmed either by transcutaneous ultrasound, or by instillation of methylene blue diluted in saline into the bladder through the Foley catheter to observe retrograde blue efflux through the stent.
- The anterior wall anastomosis is completed in a similar fashion to the posterior wall anastomosis and the redundant proximal ureter and UPJO is removed for specimen.

- Outside of double-J ureteral stents, one may elect to use externalized ureteropyelostomy stents.[31]
- Reduction pyeloplasty is rarely performed, except in cases of giant hydronephrosis that is crossing the midline. However, small amounts of redundant renal pelvis may need to be resected to avoid a mismatch and irregular closure.
- Surgical site drain is not necessary for routine, uncomplicated repairs.

Postoperative Care

Patients are typically monitored overnight after uncomplicated pyeloplasty repair. Their diet is advanced as tolerated and nonnarcotic pain control (ie, ketorolac and acetaminophen) is used. Outside of the one-time intraoperative antibiotics, no other periprocedural or prophylactic antibiotics are given. Void trial is typically performed the following morning and patients are discharged after successfully voiding and tolerating oral intake.

OUTCOMES

Robotic Anderson-Hynes dismembered pyeloplasty is associated with high levels of success (>99%) and low levels of postoperative complications (<4%) in high-volume centers.[47] Rare, but significant postoperative complications include urine leak, infection, ileus, blood transfusion, and obstruction secondary to clot or displaced stent. To ensure successful repair, follow-up imaging typically consists of ultrasounds to evaluate for stable or improved hydronephrosis. If there are no clinical symptoms of obstruction during follow-up and improved ultrasound findings, routine functional imaging is unlikely to change management and is therefore unnecessary.

SUMMARY

UPJO is a common cause of hydronephrosis in the neonatal and pediatric population that requires careful evaluation of clinical history, ultrasound, and diuretic renography. Although most patients are managed conservatively, when surgical repair is indicated it is associated with high levels of success and rare postoperative complications.

CLINICS CARE POINTS

- Congenital hydronephrosis is classified and managed based on the UTD classification scheme.

- Additional work-up with diuretic renogram should be performed in patients with significant hydronephrosis and no hydroureter to evaluate for UPJO.
- Although most patients are managed conservatively, indications for surgical repair include recurrent pain crises, differential renal function less than 40%, decline in renal function over time, urinary tract infections, worsening hydronephrosis, or nephrolithiasis.

CONFLICTS OF INTEREST

None.

REFERENCES

1. Blyth B, Snyder HM, Duckett JW. Antenatal diagnosis and subsequent management of hydronephrosis. J Urol 1993;149(4):693–8.
2. Gunn TR, Mora JD, Pease P. Antenatal diagnosis of urinary tract abnormalities by ultrasonography after 28 weeks' gestation: incidence and outcome. Am J Obstet Gynecol 1995;172(2 Pt 1):479–86.
3. Sairam S, Al-Habib A, Sasson S, et al. Natural history of fetal hydronephrosis diagnosed on midtrimester ultrasound. Ultrasound Obstet Gynecol 2001;17(3):191–6.
4. Siddique J, Lauderdale DS, VanderWeele TJ, et al. Trends in prenatal ultrasound use in the United States: 1995 to 2006. Med Care 2009;47(11): 1129–35.
5. O'Keeffe DF, Abuhamad A. Obstetric ultrasound utilization in the United States: data from various health plans. Semin Perinatol 2013;37(5):292–4.
6. Avni FE, Cos T, Cassart M, et al. Evolution of fetal ultrasonography. Eur Radiol 2007;17(2):419–31.
7. Whitworth M, Bricker L, Mullan C. Ultrasound for fetal assessment in early pregnancy. Cochrane Database Syst Rev 2015;2015(7):CD007058.
8. Grignon A, Filion R, Filiatrault D, et al. Urinary tract dilatation in utero: classification and clinical applications. Radiology 1986;160(3):645–7.
9. Fernbach SK, Maizels M, Conway JJ. Ultrasound grading of hydronephrosis: introduction to the system used by the Society for Fetal Urology. Pediatr Radiol 1993;23(6):478–80.
10. Keays MA, Guerra LA, Mihill J, et al. Reliability assessment of Society for Fetal Urology ultrasound grading system for hydronephrosis. J Urol 2008; 180(4 Suppl):1680–2 [discussion: 1682-3].
11. Zanetta VC, Rosman BM, Bromley B, et al. Variations in management of mild prenatal hydronephrosis among maternal-fetal medicine obstetricians, and pediatric urologists and radiologists. J Urol 2012; 188(5):1935–9.
12. Nguyen HT, Benson CB, Bromley B, et al. Multidisciplinary consensus on the classification of prenatal and postnatal urinary tract dilation (UTD classification system). J Pediatr Urol 2014;10(6): 982–98.
13. Lee RS, Cendron M, Kinnamon DD, et al. Antenatal hydronephrosis as a predictor of postnatal outcome: a meta-analysis. Pediatrics 2006;118(2):586–93.
14. Han M, Kim HG, Lee JD, et al. Conversion and reliability of two urological grading systems in infants: the Society for Fetal Urology and the urinary tract dilatation classifications system. Pediatr Radiol 2017;47(1):65–73.
15. Chalmers DJ, Meyers ML, Brodie KE, et al. Interrater reliability of the APD, SFU and UTD grading systems in fetal sonography and MRI. J Pediatr Urol 2016;12(5):305 e1–e305 e5.
16. Laing FC, Burke VD, Wing VW, et al. Postpartum evaluation of fetal hydronephrosis: optimal timing for follow-up sonography. Radiology 1984;152(2): 423–4.
17. Nelson CP, Lee RS, Trout AT, et al. The association of postnatal urinary tract dilation risk score with clinical outcomes. J Pediatr Urol 2019;15(4):341 e1–e341 e6.
18. Akhavan A, Shnorhavorian M, Garrison LP Jr, et al. Resource utilization and costs associated with the diagnostic evaluation of nonrefluxing primary hydronephrosis in infants. J Urol 2014;192(3):919–24.
19. Kass EJ, Majd M, Belman AB. Comparison of the diuretic renogram and the pressure perfusion study in children. J Urol 1985;134(1):92–6.
20. Shulkin BL, Mandell GA, Cooper JA, et al. Procedure guideline for diuretic renography in children 3.0. J Nucl Med Technol 2008;36(3):162–8.
21. McDaniel BB, Jones RA, Scherz H, et al. Dynamic contrast-enhanced MR urography in the evaluation of pediatric hydronephrosis: Part 2, anatomic and functional assessment of ureteropelvic junction obstruction [corrected]. AJR Am J Roentgenol 2005;185(6):1608–14.
22. Lee T, Finney E, Jha A, et al. Approaches and barriers to biomarker discovery: the example of biomarkers of renal scarring in pediatric urology. Urol Clin North Am 2023;50(1):1–17.
23. Wang HS, Cho PS, Zhi H, et al. Association between urinary biomarkers MMP-7/TIMP-2 and reduced renal function in children with ureteropelvic junction obstruction. PLoS One 2022;17(7). e0270018.
24. King LR, Coughlin PW, Bloch EC, et al. The case for immediate pyeloplasty in the neonate with ureteropelvic junction obstruction. J Urol 1984;132(4): 725–8.
25. Ulman I, Jayanthi VR, Koff SA. The long-term followup of newborns with severe unilateral hydronephrosis initially treated nonoperatively. J Urol 2000;164(3 Pt 2):1101–5.

26. Dhillon HK. Prenatally diagnosed hydronephrosis: the Great Ormond Street experience. Br J Urol 1998;81(Suppl 2):39–44.

27. Rosen S, Peters CA, Chevalier RL, et al. The kidney in congenital ureteropelvic junction obstruction: a spectrum from normal to nephrectomy. J Urol 2008;179(4):1257–63.

28. Rooks VJ, Lebowitz RL. Extrinsic ureteropelvic junction obstruction from a crossing renal vessel: demography and imaging. Pediatr Radiol 2001; 31(2):120–4.

29. Lowe FC, Marshall FF. Ureteropelvic junction obstruction in adults. Urology 1984;23(4):331–5.

30. Mitterberger M, Pinggera GM, Neururer R, et al. Comparison of contrast-enhanced color Doppler imaging (CDI), computed tomography (CT), and magnetic resonance imaging (MRI) for the detection of crossing vessels in patients with ureteropelvic junction obstruction (UPJO). Eur Urol 2008;53(6): 1254–60.

31. Gopal M, Peycelon M, Caldamone A, et al. Management of ureteropelvic junction obstruction in children-a roundtable discussion. J Pediatr Urol 2019;15(4):322–9.

32. Anderson JC, Hynes W. Retrocaval ureter; a case diagnosed pre-operatively and treated successfully by a plastic operation. Br J Urol 1949;21(3):209–14.

33. Peters CA, Schlussel RN, Retik AB. Pediatric laparoscopic dismembered pyeloplasty. J Urol 1995; 153(6):1962–5.

34. Rabinovitch HH. Renal operation in children via a posterior approach. J Urol 1981;125(1):61–2.

35. Orland SM, Snyder HM, Duckett JW. The dorsal lumbotomy incision in pediatric urological surgery. J Urol 1987;138(4 Pt 2):963–6.

36. Das S, Egan RM, Amar AD. Dorsal lumbotomy for surgery of the upper urinary tract. J Urol 1987; 137(5):862–4.

37. Braga LH, Lorenzo AJ, Bagli DJ, et al. Comparison of flank, dorsal lumbotomy and laparoscopic approaches for dismembered pyeloplasty in children older than 3 years with ureteropelvic junction obstruction. J Urol 2010;183(1):306–11.

38. Liu DB, Ellimoottil C, Flum AS, et al. Contemporary national comparison of open, laparoscopic, and robotic-assisted laparoscopic pediatric pyeloplasty. J Pediatr Urol 2014;10(4):610–5.

39. Varda BK, Wang Y, Chung BI, et al. Has the robot caught up? National trends in utilization, perioperative outcomes, and cost for open, laparoscopic, and robotic pediatric pyeloplasty in the United States from 2003 to 2015. J Pediatr Urol 2018; 14(4):336 e1–e336 e8.

40. Avery DI, Herbst KW, Lendvay TS, et al. Robot-assisted laparoscopic pyeloplasty: multi-institutional experience in infants. J Pediatr Urol 2015;11(3): 139 e1–e5.

41. Rague JT, Shannon R, Rosoklija I, et al. Robot-assisted laparoscopic urologic surgery in infants weighing </=10 kg: a weight stratified analysis. J Pediatr Urol 2021;17(6):857 e1–e857 e7.

42. Corbett HJ, Mullassery D. Outcomes of endopyelotomy for pelviureteric junction obstruction in the paediatric population: a systematic review. J Pediatr Urol 2015;11(6):328–36.

43. Smith TW Jr, Wang X, Singer MA, et al. Enhanced recovery after surgery: a clinical review of implementation across multiple surgical subspecialties. Am J Surg 2020;219(3):530–4.

44. Cockrell SN, Hendren WH. The importance of visualizing the ureter before performing a pyeloplasty. J Urol 1990;144(2 Pt 2):588–92 [discussion: 593-4].

45. Rushton HG, Salem Y, Belman AB, et al. Pediatric pyeloplasty: is routine retrograde pyelography necessary? J Urol 1994;152(2 Pt 2):604–6.

46. Gargollo PC. Hidden incision endoscopic surgery: description of technique, parental satisfaction and applications. J Urol 2011;185(4):1425–31.

47. Silay MS, Spinoit AF, Undre S, et al. Global minimally invasive pyeloplasty study in children: Results from the Pediatric Urology Expert Group of the European Association of Urology Young Academic Urologists working party. J Pediatr Urol 2016;12(4):229 e1–e7.

Embryology, Treatment, and Outcomes of Ureteroceles in Children

Hans G. Pohl, MD

KEYWORDS

• Ureterocele • Orthotopic • Ectopic • Duplex system • Single system

KEY POINTS

- The position of ureteral orifice correlates with function of associated renal moiety.
- Ureteroceles associated with good renal function and prompt drainage or ureteroceles associated with no renal function can be managed nonoperatively.
- Endoscopic puncture of ureteroceles addresses most cases; iatrogenic reflux may rarely require secondary surgery.
- Robot-assisted laparoscopic upper pole nephroureterectomy and ureteroureterostomy procedures are rarely associated with complications.

INTRODUCTION

To my knowledge, this is the fourth chapter of the Urologic Clinics of North America devoted to the management of ureteroceles, and I would like to begin by acknowledging the contributions of prior authors, particularly Timberlake and Corbett who provided the most recent and comprehensive issue from which I borrow heavily, updating theirs with data published since 2014.[1–3]

A ureterocele is a congenital cystic dilatation of the intravesical ureter that may affect either a single system kidney or the upper pole of a duplex system. Chwalla's hypothesis from 1927 remains the most often quoted.[4] He postulated that during normal development, the distal ureter is occluded by a membrane composed of urogenital sinus tissue and ureteric epithelium, ureteroceles being caused by failure of this membrane to dissolve. However, the routinely present duplex collecting system, the association with upper pole ureters, the presence of defects in ureteral muscle and renal parenchyma, the variable insertion along the course of Wolffian duct migration, and the rare presence of gaping ureterocele orifices, all suggest a more complex embryologic origin (**Fig. 1**).[5] It is this disordered embryology that must be understood to select optimal treatment (**Table 1**).

Stenotic ureteroceles are the most common type associated with single and duplicated systems. The stenotic orifice may be located on the trigone, on the upside or on the downside—as viewed endoscopically—of the dilated ureterocele. Most kidneys associated with single-system ureteroceles have preserved function, whereas most upper pole moieties associated with ureteroceles have reduced function. Stenotic ureteroceles occupying an intravesical location do not generally obstruct the bladder neck if sessile. However, pedunculated stenotic ureteroceles may impede bladder emptying.

Sphincteric ureteroceles traverse submucosally beyond a trigonal insertion and cross the bladder neck, terminating in the urethra anywhere from the internal sphincter to just beyond the external sphincter. The trans-sphincteric portion is usually of normal caliber but may also be as dilated as the ureterocele itself. In fact, the presence of ureterocele dilation is dictated by where the orifice terminates in the urethra; dilated ureteroceles

Urology and Pediatrics, The George Washington University School of Medicine and Health Sciences, Urology, Children's National Hospital, 111 Michigan Avenue, NW, Suite WW-4400, Washington, DC 20010, USA
E-mail address: hpohl@childrensnational.org

Urol Clin N Am 50 (2023) 371–389
https://doi.org/10.1016/j.ucl.2023.04.007

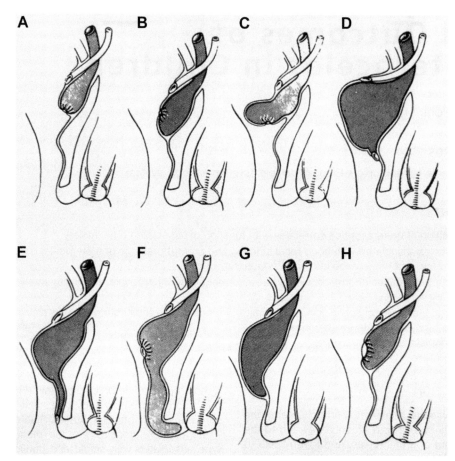

Fig. 1. Types of ureteroceles located on the ectopic ureter of duplex systems, showing also the anatomic relation of the expansion to the orifice. (*A, B, C*) Stenotic ureteroceles: terminal expansions with orifice raised off the trigone (*A*), perched on the dome (*B*), and underhung (*C*). (*D, E*) Sphincteric ureteroceles: subterminal expansion, with the orifice, large or small, resting on the posterior wall of the urethra. (*F*) Cecoureterocele: terminal expansion with long drawn-out caudal extension forming a "cecum" in the submucosal plane of the urethra. (*G*) Blind ureterocele. (*H*) Nonobstructed ureterocele: terminal expansion with large orifice lying within the confines of the bladder. (*From* Stephens, FD (1971), Cecoureterocele and concepts on the embryology etiology of ureteroceles. Aust N.Z. J. Surg. 40:239, see **Fig 1**.)

form more commonly when the orifice is within the internal sphincter, rather than distal to it.[6] In fact, the orifice of a sphincteric ureterocele is generally not stenotic but wide, obstruction being caused by constriction of the internal sphincter at rest. Thus, when the bladder empties during voiding, so does the sphincteric ureterocele. By comparison to the lateral placement of stenotic ureteroceles, sphincteric ureteroceles occupy both lateral and central portions of the trigone.

Stephens, observing peristaltic activity in some single-system stenotic ureteroceles, used a variety of procedures to treat single-system ureteroceles without creating vesicoureteral reflux (VUR). Nine of sixteen patients with stenotic ureteroceles underwent enlargement and partial excision or incision of the orifice, 7 of whom showed no VUR

on follow-up, in support of the notion that the distal ureter remains sufficiently competent in some to function as a nonrefluxing valve.[7] *Sphincterostenotic ureteroceles* follow the same pathway as sphincteric ureteroceles, however, with stenotic orifices. Thus, they are obstructed both by the narrow orifice as well as by the bladder neck. Dilatation of the ureterocele is sufficient to obstruct the bladder neck.

Cecoureteroceles generally have orifices within the bladder located on the upside of the ureterocele but also has a long tongue of distended distal ureter traversing from the trigone through the bladder neck and into the urethra. The orifice may be stenotic or widely patent. Cecoureteroceles with stenotic orifices fill from the renal moiety only, whereas open orifices fill from the bladder.

Table 1
Classification of duplex ureteroceles, with clinical correlates

Ureterocele	Frequency[a] N (%)	Features
Intravesical		
Stenotic	25 (42)	Small ureteral orifice obstructing the upper pole
Nonobstructed	3 (5)	Large ureteral orifice without obstruction
Extravesical		
Sphincteric	21 (35)	The orifice opens outside the bladder and the ureterocele extends into the bladder neck and urethra. The orifice is normal or large and opens proximal to the external sphincter. In women the meatus may open beyond the external sphincter. The bladder neck obstructs the upper pole, as it is contracted at rest.
Sphincterostenotic	4 (7)	Similar to sphincteric but with an obstructed orifice.
Ceco	3 (5)	The orifice opens inside the bladder, but a blind pouch extends into the bladder neck and urethra. The pouch fills on voiding that obstructs urine flow.
Blind ectopic	3 (5)	Similar to sphincteric but with no ureteral orifice.

[a] One ureterocele was unclassified.
Adapted from Stephens (2002) and Docimo, Canning, Khoury (2007).

Blind ureteroceles extend over the trigone and into the bladder neck. Bladder neck obstruction is uniformly seen.

Ureteroceles have been identified in up to 1 in 500 autopsy specimens and occur 4 times more frequently in women than men. Ureteroceles are associated with duplicated collecting systems in 95% of women, but they are associated with single collecting systems in 66% of men. Eighty percent of ureteroceles are associated with the upper pole of a duplicated collecting system, and the remainder are associated with single systems. Single-system ureteroceles more commonly occur on the left side. Eighty-five percent of ureteroceles are unilateral. Nearly all occur in Whites.[8–12] VUR is seen into 17% of ureteroceles themselves, into 54% of ipsilateral lower pole ureters, and into 28% of contralateral lower pole ureters of duplex systems. Among single-system ureteroceles, VUR is seen into 9% of both the ipsilateral and contralateral ureters[12] (**Table 2**).

SURGICAL INDICATIONS AND OPTIONS

Ureteroceles have been associated with several upper and lower urinary tract anatomic abnormalities that influence the type and timing of management (see **Table 2**). The tenets of pediatric urologic management include the following: (1) preservation of renal function; (2) avoidance of recurrent, symptomatic urinary tract infection; (3) urinary continence; and (4) optimizing quality of life through judicious application of imaging as well as nonoperative and surgical treatment (**Box 1** and **2**).

Several approaches have been applied for ureterocele management, consensus being stymied by small sample sizes and heterogeneity of anatomic findings among patient populations and inconsistency in outcomes measured. The incidence of febrile urinary tract infection (fUTI), presence and degree of VUR, upper pole dysfunction, and ureteral and/or bladder dysfunction are variables that can be taken into consideration. The most common outcome measured is the rate of secondary procedures following initial management. However, a surgeon's bias often is difficult to decode. In an editorial, Grahame Smith commented that studies "measured what the surgeon indications were for surgery in this condition, rather than what caused illness in the patient" and that "good outcome measures would be

Table 2
Anatomic problems associated with ureteroceles

Upper Pole Moiety	Lower Pole Moiety	Bladder Neck/Urethra
Ipsilateral VUR	Ipsilateral VUR	Obstruction
Ipsilateral obstruction	Contralateral VUR	Urethral prolapse
Poor or nonfunction	—	—

Box 1
Goals of therapy for children with ureterocele

1. Preservation of renal function
   - Upper pole moiety
   - Lower pole moiety
2. Prevention of recurrent, symptomatic infection
3. Elimination of clinically significant vesicoureteral reflux
4. Relief of ureteral obstruction
5. Relieve of bladder and urethral obstruction
6. Preservation of urinary continence

Adapted from Timberlake M.D. and Corbett S.T. Urol Clin N Am 42(2015) 61–76.

---

incidence of [UTIs], prevention of renal injury, [and] maintenance of continence."[13]

Historically, a single-stage open reconstruction entailed upper pole nephroureterectomy (UPPN) combined with excision of the ureterocele, ureteral reimplantation (single- or common-sheath), and reconstruction of the bladder base and outlet, as indicated. Surgeons have since considered the necessity of upper and lower urinary tract reconstruction, favoring either isolated upper tract or isolated lower tract approaches first. As for other conditions, open surgery has been supplanted by minimally invasive approaches, whether laparoscopic or robot-assisted.

I have organized this review by focusing first on the upper urinary tract and next the lower urinary tract, setting the narrative with a discussion of expectations for renal function at baseline and what may be achievable without surgery.

EXPECTATIONS FOR UPPER MOIETY RENAL FUNCTION AND INFLUENCE ON NONOPERATIVE MANAGEMENT OF URETEROCELES

FD Stephens should be credited for correlating the embryology of upper and lower urinary tract development with clinically observed phenomena (**Fig. 2**). Ureteral bud position on the Wolffian duct not only determines the final location of the ureteral orifice but also the fate of the metanephric blastema and, thus, whether renal dysplasia is present and to what degree.

Among duplex kidneys, the upper pole provides only up to 33% of that kidney's contribution to total renal function or up to 16% of overall renal function. Pathologic examination of UPPN specimens

has found irreversible changes in up to 92% of specimens.[14] Given the upper pole's marginal contribution to total renal function, it seems illogical to pursue extreme measures to save it when associated with a congenital anomaly such as a ureterocele.

Indeed, renal function is affected in 74% of upper poles associated with ureteroceles and in 20% of single systems associated with ureteroceles.[12] Affected upper poles generally contribute between 4% and 8% of total renal function. On average, efforts to preserve the upper pole result in a gain of up to 2.25% of total renal function from endoscopic incision and 2.25 ± 2.34% following upper pole salvage,[14,15] whereas UPPN on average results in a 1.25 ± 2.7% reduction in overall function.[14]

The upper pole moiety's often meager contribution to renal function has led some to consider whether no procedure is justified under certain circumstances, some ureteroceles being asymptomatic. Although only 4 studies encompassing 45 patients have focused on this concept, these limited data support nonoperative management (**Table 3**). Patients who have nonfunctioning or poorly functioning renal moieties and no evidence of high-grade obstruction on diuresis renography, regardless of VUR status, are candidates for a nonoperative approach, at least initially. Borrowing from the modern management of VUR, surgery is reserved for those suffering breakthrough

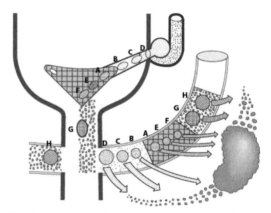

Fig. 2. The correlation between position of the ureteral orifice and expected renal function. Ureteral buds that emit from an ideal position on the Wolffian duct penetrate the midzone of the metanephric blastema, which elicits proper reciprocal induction between the ureter and kidney. A more cephalad position (G, H) or more caudad position (B, C, D) on the Wolffian duct result in ureteral orifices that are more caudad or cephalad within the lower genitourinary tract. (*From* The Kelalis-King-Belman Textbook of Clinical Pediatric Urology, 6th Edition.)

Table 3
Outcome of renal moieties nonoperatively managed

Author, Year	N	SSU or DSU (N)	Nonfunctioning (N, %)	Mean UP Function (%)	Outcomes/Comments
Shankar et al,[19] 2001	52	DSU (52)	14 (26.9)	<10	At baseline, VUR grade 1(2), grade 2 (4), and grade 3 (2). No patient with fUTI in follow-up. VUR resolved spontaneously in 3 out of 4 studied.
Coplen and Austin,[38] 2004	8	SSU (4) DSU (4)	SSU (4 MCDK) DSU (4 MCDK)	0	At baseline, VUR grade 2 (1 ipsilateral LP, 1 contralateral) and grade 3 (1 ipsilateral LP and contralateral grade 2 in same patient). Only 1 fUTI in the patient with bilateral VUR. VUR resolved in 2 out of 2 patients studied. Hydronephrosis improved (3) or stable (5).
Han et al,[16] 2005	13	SSU (2) DSU (11)	SSU (2 MCDK) DSU (1 MCDK) DSU (0)	0 40.8 (28–65)	9 out of 13 patients did not undergo surgery having demonstrated no risk for fUTI, involution of MCCDK (2), stable nonfunctioning upper pole without hydronephrosis (1), and functioning UP with improvement in hydronephrosis (6). VUR, present in 5 out of 6 LP systems at baseline, resolved in all.
Direnna and Leonard,[20] 2006	10	SSU (4) DSU (6)	SSU (1 MCDK)	"Functioning" but not quantified (6)	All SSUs were orthotopic, and all DSUs were ectopic. Hydronephrosis resolved (5), improved by 1 SFU grade (2) or stable (2).

fUTIs or with high-grade hydronephrosis in follow-up.[16–20] (**Box 2**).

Box 2
Candidates for nonoperative management of ureteroceles

1 SSU or DSU, ectopic or orthotopic AND

2 Good or absent function in ureterocele moiety AND

3 Absence of grade IV or V VUR AND

4 Absence of high-grade obstruction by diuresis renography AND

5 Absence of BOO

Adapted from Timberlake M.D. and Corbett S.T. Urol Clin N Am 42(2015) 61–76.

UPPER TRACT APPROACH: UPPER POLE NEPHRECTOMY AND HIGH URETEROURETEROSTOMY/URETEROPYELOSTOMY

Upper tract approaches include renal salvage by ureteroureterostomy (UU) or ureteropyelostomy (UP) or removal of the upper pole and most of its subtending ureter by UPPN. Open and minimally invasive approaches yield equivalent resolution of upper pole hydronephrosis and reduction of risk for recurrent UTI. Neither approach is without complications, though.[14,21] Although UU/UP may result in anastomotic strictures and UPPN may result in partial or complete loss of lower pole function, urine leaks may occur following either.[14,21] Overall, minimally invasive approaches offer a reduction in blood loss, postoperative pain, and length of stay as compared with open surgery. Summaries of the rates of complications following transperitoneal or retroperitoneal access for laparoscopic or robot-assisted laparoscopic UPPN as well as UU and of operative times are provided[22,23] (**Tables 4 and 5, Boxes 3–5**).

Vates and colleagues compared the rate of adjunct surgery, postoperative UTIs, and change in differential renal function among 43 children (56% of whom presented with rUTI) undergoing either UU/UP (n = 12) or UPPN (n = 31).[14] UU/UP was performed for ureterocele (6), ectopic ureter (3), VUR (1), and unknown reason (2), whereas UPPN was performed for ureterocele (11), ectopic ureter (19), and VUR (1). Preoperative and postoperative nuclear renograms were available in 8 children who underwent UU/UP and 8 children who underwent UPPN. There was no statistically significant difference in the preoperative versus postoperative renal function or the rates of adjunct surgery or UTI

between patients undergoing salvage by UU/UP or UPPN.

Esposito and colleagues have shown in a multi-institutional cohort of children who underwent either laparoscopic intraperitoneal UPPN (52) or retroperitoneoscopic UPPN (50) that retroperitoneoscopic UPPN carries a greater risk for complications, such as urinoma, retained distal stump, and lower collecting system injury, in addition to longer operative time and hospitalization.[24] However, their findings are refuted by 2 additional series demonstrating a low risk of complications following retroperitoneoscopic approach.

Joyeux and colleagues performed retroperitoneoscopic UPPN in 25 patients with nonfunctioning upper pole moieties associated with ureterocele (n = 11) or ectopia associated with incontinence (n = 6) or hydronephrosis (n = 8).[23] Postoperatively, all children underwent sonography and 99m-Tc-DMSA renal scans that identified partial loss of lower pole function in 17% but complete loss of function was never seen.[23] Subsequently, MacDonald and colleagues reviewed their series of 173 minimally invasive total nephrectomies (119) and heminephrectomies (54) done via transperitoneal or retroperitoneal approaches. Overall, 7 (4%) patients underwent conversion to open and 19.6% underwent further surgery, including 8 distal ureteral stumps that were removed. Among those having a retroperitoneoscopic approach, 1.9% underwent conversion to open and 13.1% underwent further surgery. In their hands, retroperitoneoscopic surgery was not associated with an increased risk for surgery.

Neheman and colleagues compared 4 different surgical approaches for UPPN of a nonfunctioning moiety, including open UPPN (n = 24), laparoscopic UPPN (n = 7), robotic UPPN (n = 18), and laparoscopic single-site UPPN (n = 10).[22] Open UPPN was associated with higher median estimated blood loss, higher analgesic requirement (narcotic and nonnarcotic), longer hospital stay, and more use of drains, than minimally invasive approaches (**Table 6**).

Pooling data from 11 series of laparoscopic intraperitoneal UPPN and 9 series of retroperitoneoscopic UPPN suggest that intraperitoneal surgery outperforms retroperitoneoscopic surgery narrowly in terms of open conversion (0.3% vs 5%, respectively), urinoma or leak (4.2% vs 4%, respectively), stump infection (1.5% vs 5%, respectively), and partial or complete renal loss (3.9% vs 3%, respectively) (see **Table 4**). Although most complications can be managed in a straightforward manner, partial or complete loss of renal function is a difficult outcome to accept and one that may be avoidable through avoidance of

Table 4
Perioperative complications reported with minimally invasive and open upper pole nephroureterectomy

Approach	N	Open Conversion (%)	Urinoma or Leak (%)	Stump Infection (%)	Renal Loss[a] (%)
Laparoscopic Intraperitoneal UPPN					
Chertin et al, 2007	10	1 (10)	0	0	0
Denes et al, 2007	19	0	0	3 (15.7)	0
Garcia-Aparicio et al, 2010	9	0	0	0	0
You et al,[21] 2010	17	0	1 (5.8)	1 (5.8)	0
Abedinzadeh et al,[49] 2012	14	0	0	0	1 (7.1)
Cabezali et al,[50] 2013	28	0	2 (7.1)	0	2 (7.1)
Dingemann et al,[51] 2013	20	0	1 (5)	0	0
Golebiewski et al,[52] 2013	15	0	0	0	0
Esposito et al,[24] 2015	52	0	8 (15.3)	2 (3.8)	0
Marte et al,[53] 2015	22	0	1 (4.5)	0	0
Szklarz et al,[54] 2021	130	0	1 (0.7)	0	10 (17)
Total	*336*	*1 (0.3)*	*14 (4.2)*	*5 (1.5)*	*13 (3.9)*
Laparoscopic Retroperitoneal UPPN					
Valla et al, 2003	24	3 (12.5)	3 (12.5)	0	0
Lee et al,[33] 2005	14	0	1 (7.1)	0	0
Wallis et al, 2006	22	4 (18.1)	3 (13.6)	0	2 (9.1)
Jayram et al, 2011	142	11 (7.7)	7 (4.9)	1 (0.7)	7 (4.9)
Chen et al,[55] 2014	31	0	0	0	0
Esposito et al,[24] 2015	50	3 (6)	6 (12)	8 (16)	0
Joyeux et al,[23] 2017	25	0	2 (8)	2 (8)	4 (17)
MacDonald et al,[56] 2019	160	3 (1.9)	1 (0.6)	8 (5)	1 (0.6)
Wadham et al,[57] 2021	56	0	0	5 (8.9)	4 (7.1)
Total	*524*	*24 (5)*	*23 (4)*	*24 (5)*	*18 (3)*
Robotic Retroperitoneal UPPN					
Olsen & Jorgensen, 2005	14	2 (14.2)	0	1 (7.1)	0
Total	*14*	*2 (14.2)*	*0*	*1 (7.1)*	*0*
Robotic Intraperitoneal UPPN					
Lee et al, 2009	9	0	1 (11.1)	0	0
Mason et al, 2014	21	0	0	0	0
Malik et al, 2015	16	0	2 (13)	2 (13)	0
Total	*46*	*0*	*3 (6.5)*	*2 (4.3)*	*0*
Open Retroperitoneal UPPN (Dorsal Lumbotomy)					
Roshan et al, 2020[58]	50	N.A.	0	0	1 (2)
Total	*50*	*N.A.*	*0*	*0*	*1 (2)*
Robotic Intraperitoneal UU					
Gonzalez and Piaggi, 2007	5	0	0	0	0
Leavitt et al, 2012	8	0	0	0	0
Kawal et al,[31] 2019 (<10% UP function	25	0	0	0	0
Kawal et al,[31] 2019 (>10% UP function	15	0	0	0	0
Total	*53*	*0*	*0*	*0*	*0*

[a] Complete or partial renal loss.
Adapted from Timberlake M.D. and Corbett S.T. Urol Clin N Am 42(2015) 61 to 76.

Table 5
Operative duration for alternate minimally invasive heminephrectomy approaches

Approach	Mean Duration (min)
Laparoscopic Intraperitoneal UPPN	
Chertin et al, 2007	NR
Denes et al, 2007	147
Garcia-Aparicio et al, 2010	182
You et al, 2010	167
Cabezali et al, 2013	137
Esposito et al, 2015[24]	166[a]
Marte et al, 2015[53]	154
Laparoscopic Retroperitoneal UPPN	
Valla et al, 2003	300
Lee et al, 2005	194
Wallis et al, 2006	174
Jayram et al, 2011	120
Esposito et al, 2015[24]	255[a]
Robot-assisted Retroperitoneal UPPN	
Olsen & Jorgensen, 2005	176
Robot-assisted Intraperitoneal UPPN	
Lee et al, 2009	275
Mason et al, 2014	300
Robot-assisted Intraperitoneal UU	
Gonzalez and Piaggi, 2007	257
Leavitt et al, 2012	227
Kawal et al, 2019[b]	170[a]
Kawal et al, 2019[c]	200[a]

[a] Median.
[b] (Subgroup with <10% UP function).
[c] (Subgroup with >10% UP function).
Adapted from Timberlake M.D. and Corbett S.T. Urol Clin N Am 42(2015) 61 to 76.

traction on the lower pole and careful dissection around the upper pole, taking into consideration the often-anomalous blood supply in duplex kidneys[25] (**Fig. 4**).

UPPER TRACT APPROACH: UPPER POLE URETERAL CLIPPING

In 2014, Romao and colleagues described their earliest experience with laparoscopic ureteral ligation of the ectopic ureter associated with nonfunctioning upper pole moieties. The initial cohort of 9 girls with urinary incontinence became dry and were asymptomatic at longest follow-up of 27 months; even 8 girls developed some degree of

Box 3
Operative technique for laparoscopic heminephrectomy (laparoscopic or robot-assisted) with partial ureterectomy

1. Optional. Cystoscopy with retrograde pyeloureterogram to define the surgical anatomy. Ureteral catheterization is occasionally performed for intraoperative identification of the ureter draining the functional pole.

2. A Foley catheter is placed.

   a. The ureteral stent is either internalized to the Foley drainage bag or drained separately.

3. The patient is positioned in a 45° modified flank position.

   a. Three ports are placed. A camera port (8.5 mm or 12 mm) is placed near the umbilicus followed by insufflation of the abdomen. Two instrument ports (5 mm or 8 mm) are placed (**Fig. 3**). An additional 5 mm port for liver retraction can be placed in the left midclavicular line for right-sided cases.

   b. The robot is docked.

4. The colon is reflected medially and both duplex system ureters are identified medial to the iliopsoas muscle on the affected side.

5. In UPPN, great care should be taken to avoid injury to the inferior pole vasculature as it crosses anterior to the superior moiety ureter (Video 1).

   a. The dilated nonfunctioning ureter is divided proximally allowing decompression of the dilated moiety. In UPPN, the divided proximal upper pole ureter is passed beneath the lower moiety vasculature. (Video 2) The ureter is used to facilitate retraction and mobilization of the affected moiety.

   b. The demarcation between the functioning and nonfunctioning moieties is visualized and divided using diathermy or LigaSure (Medtronic, Minneapolis, MN, USA) or Ethicon Harmonic (Johnson&Johnson, Irvine, CA, USA). (Video 3)

   c. The superior moiety ureter is dissected as far distally as possible and then divided. If the divided ureter is known to be refluxing, the stump can be oversewn with absorbable suture. For this, the 0 PDS Ethicon Endoloop Ligature (Johnson&Johnson, Irvine, CA, USA) is useful. If the ureter is nonrefluxing, the stump is left open. (Video 4)

   d. The specimens are removed through the umbilical port incision.

Adapted from Timberlake M.D. and Corbett S.T. Urol Clin N Am 42(2015) 61 to 76.

upper pole hydronephrosis.[26] This same group extended the indications for clipping, reporting their observations on 35 consecutive patients (23 women, 12 men) with (1) duplex system with ectopic ureter (45.7%), (2) duplex system with a large ureterocele (11.4%), (3) other duplex system (8.6%), and (4) single-system kidneys (34.3%). After a median $\pm$ standard deviation follow-up of

20.8 $\pm$ 13.8 months (interquartile range 8.5–30, range 6–50) 97.2% of the patients remained asymptomatic, and only 1 patient underwent an additional procedure—laparoscopic nephrectomy—for pyonephrosis.[27] Although clipping is not expected to resolve upper pole hydronephrosis, it seems to be of no consequence to patients so long as the ectopic ureter is no longer in continuity with the lower urinary tract.[27,28]

LOWER TRACT APPROACH: URETEROURETEROSTOMY

The criteria that have traditionally been applied in selecting UU include good upper pole function, absence of lower pole VUR, and comparable caliber of the upper and lower pole ureters. However, some have shown that these requirements do not need to be met for UU to be successful, particularly in light of how rarely the upper pole contributes a clinically impactful amount of renal function.[29,30] Advocates of lower tract UUs cite a lower incidence of symptoms associated with the ureteral stumps that result from UPPN and upper tract UU/UP. Open and laparoscopic approaches have been used, but increasingly robot-assisted laparoscopic UU is chosen.

Kawal and colleagues assessed whether the degree of upper pole function influence surgical outcomes in 53 children undergoing open (13) or robot-assisted UU (40). Patients were segregated by upper pole function greater than 10% (7 open and 25 robot-assisted) versus less than 10% (6 open and 15 robot-assisted).[31] The rate of postoperative complications, need for adjunct surgery, and radiological outcomes were no different between the 2 groups.[31]

Biles and colleagues reported a 100% success rate in achieving resolution of upper pole hydronephrosis in 12 children with duplex systems and ureteral ectopia, none of whom had coincidental lower pole VUR.[32]

McLeod and colleagues performed UU on 41 patients (43 renal units) with ureterocele (n = 17), ectopic ureter (25), or triplication (n = 1). In 36 patients UU was performed alone, whereas in 5 UU was performed with excision of ureterocele and lower pole reimplantation. UU was performed as an initial approach in 11 patients, whereas it was the secondary procedure performed in 6 patients after failed endoscopic puncture. Size disparity between the upper and lower ureters was addressed by open or laparoscopic ureteral tapering. The median upper pole relative function was characterized in 24/43 patients as 17% (range, 0%–35%); 0% in 6 patients, less than 15% in 10 patients, and greater than 15% in 8.

Table 6
Comparison of 4 methods of upper pole nephroureterectomy

	OPN (n = 24)	LPN (n = 7)	RPN (n = 18)	LESS-PN (n = 10)	P
Patient characteristics and demographics					
Median age, months (IQR)	14.5 (10.5–24.2	11.7 (6.7–4.0	43.9 (17–131.5	12.9 (8.9–16.1	.100
Median weight, kg (IQR)	11.4 (9–13.7	9.2 (7.1–10.6	14.4 (9.9–32.8	9.45 (8.7–10.4	.187
Sex (M/F)	12/12	1/6	5/13	1/9	.115
Surgery side (R/L)	13/11	1/6	8/10	5/5	.381
Resected pole (upper/lower)	18/6	7/0	15/3	9/1	.487
Perioperative data					
Median operative time, min (range)	154.5 (108–413	190 (159–355)	256 (163–458)	140 (65–245)	.005
Median EBL, cc (range)	10 (0–125)	5 (0–50)	5 (0–100)	5 (0–20)	.013
Use of drains (%)	70.8	57.1	22.2	0	.015
Urinary catheter (%)	91.7	85.7	77.8	50	.088
Median LOS, days (range)	3 (2–24)	1 (1–2)	2 (1–4)	1 (1–1)	.005
Postoperative analgesic use					
Median ibuprofen mg/kg/d (range)	0.5 (0–60)	0	0.3 (0–41.88)	0.1 (0–10.24)	.186
Median acetaminophen mg/kg/d (range)	72.12 (0–209)	35.78 (30–47.7)	43.90 (19.9–195)	34.9 (20–45.18)	.004
Median ketorolac mg/kg/d (range)	0	0.50 (0–1.53)	0.52 (0–2.53)	1.01 0–1.53)	.005
Median morphine equivalents mg/kg/d (range)	0.554 (0.03–6.13)	0.015 (0–0.07)	0.039 (0–0.42)	0	.005

Abbreviations: EBL, estimated blood loss; IQR, interquartile range; LOS, length of stay.
Adapted from Neheman A et al. Urology. Mar 2019;125:196 to 201.

Only 2 complications were seen, one stricture of the ureterovesical junction obstruction at the reimplanted segment and one anastomotic stricture of the UU.

Significant size disparity between upper and lower pole ureters may be best managed by lower UU rather than higher approaches in order to minimize the length of ureteral stump available that may result in symptomatic urinary tract infection in up to 12% of patients.[33]

LOWER TRACT APPROACH: URETEROCELE EXCISION AND URETERAL REIMPLANTATION

Ureterocele excision with reconstruction of the bladder floor and ureteral reimplantation (single system or common sheath) is less frequently performed but remains part of the pediatric urologist's toolkit. Lower tract reconstruction is considered challenging for the following reasons: (1) significant ureteral dilatation made more challenging in the context of the duplex system where there is a size discrepancy between the 2 ureters, (2) disruption of the detrusor of the bladder floor, (3) encroachment on the bladder neck and proximal urethra, and (4) possible need to manage contralateral VUR as well in a small bladder. A variety of techniques have been described, which are worthy of review here.

Yamazaki and colleagues demonstrated in 2 children a technique for in situ plication of the dilated upper pole ureter with concomitant common sheath reimplantation when the diameter of the common sheath measures greater than 18 mm[34] (Fig. 5). The upper tracts were successfully decompressed in both patients. However, although upper tract decompression is achievable, the frequent criticism of lower tract

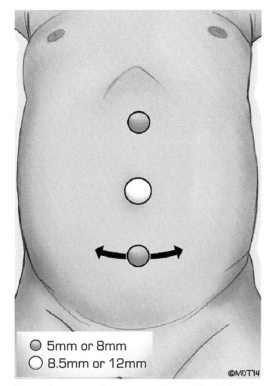

Fig. 3. Placement of laparoscopic ports for infant surgery. Three ports are placed. A camera port (8.5 mm or 12 mm) is placed near the umbilicus followed by insufflation of the abdomen. Two instrument ports (5 mm or 8 mm) are placed.

○ 5mm or 8mm
○ 8.5mm or 12mm
©MDT'14

reconstruction is that surgery at the bladder base and neck results in incontinence. De Jong and colleagues addressed this in a review of 40 patients who underwent primary lower tract reconstruction. Among female patients, the ectopic ureterocele opened in the bladder neck (5), proximal urethra (9), distal urethra (5), and vulva (9), whereas it opened into the prostatic urethra in 9 male patients. Secondary endoscopic procedures were done in 32.5% for persistent reflux (n = 9) and obstructive voiding (n = 4). Although all patients were continent in follow-up, 11 (27.5%) of the patients had dysfunctional voiding with urodynamically measured bladder capacity on average of 124% of expected capacity for age.[35]

Beanović and colleagues similarly reported a 94% continence rate during a median follow-up of 9.6 years, during which 17% of the patients had 1 to 2 uncomplicated UTIs. Secondary endoscopic procedures were performed in 31.5% for persistent VUR (n = 10) and obstructive voiding (n = 7). Biofeedback training was offered to 11 patients (20.3%) for dysfunctional voiding.[36]

More recently, Ting and colleagues reported a means to perform lower urinary tract reconstruction in young infants while avoiding complex excision of the ureterocele and repair of the bladder floor[37] (**Fig. 6**). In their series, 32 patients with ectopic duplex system ureteroceles (DSUs) underwent the "in-and-out" bladder approach at a median age of 7.8 months (range: 1.5–36 months), some undergoing the procedure only 14 days after

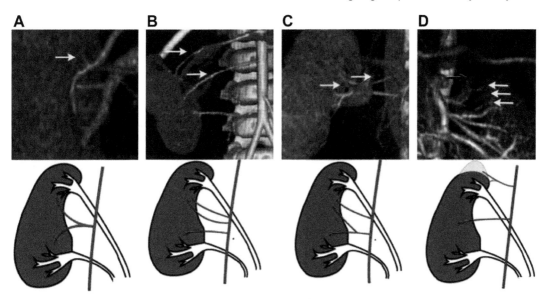

Fig. 4. Computed tomography angiography and illustrations of vascular variations in 84 duplex kidneys. (*A*) One branch (*yellow arrow*) of the renal artery supplies the upper pole (73.1%). (*B*) Two accessory renal arteries (*yellow arrow*) supply the upper pole simultaneously (19.4%). (*C*) One branch of the renal artery and one accessory renal artery (*yellow arrow*) supply the upper pole (4.3%). (*D*) Branches (*yellow arrow*) of the adrenal artery (*blue arrow*) supply the upper pole (1.1%). (*Adapted from* Luo J et al. *J Pediatr Surg*. Oct 2019;54(10):2130 to 2133.)

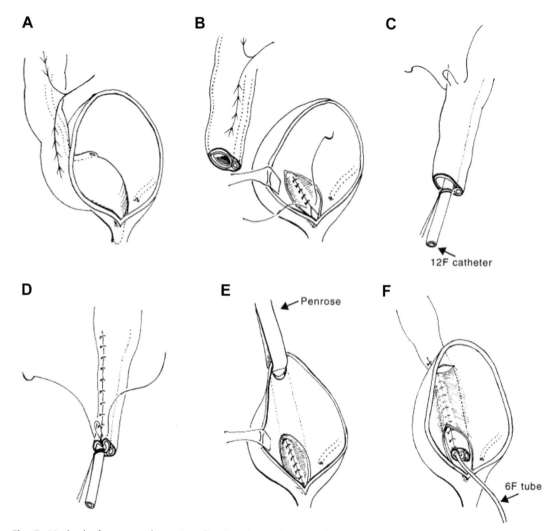

Fig. 5. Method of upper pole ureter plication during lower urinary tract reconstruction. (*A*) Excise common sheath and ureterocele, keeping blood supply undisturbed. Complete downward dissection of the ureterocele should be performed to avoid leaving a lip of incised ureterocele. (*B*) The detrusor muscle is closed using interrupted 3-0 polyglactin sutures to reinforce the insufficient detrusor backing. (*C*) When the diameter is greater than 18 mm, proceed with the common sheath ureteral plication over a 12-Fr catheter into the upper pole ureter. (*D*) 5-0 Polydioxanone sutures are placed in an inverting Lembert fashion, 5 mm apart, through the wall of the common ureteral sheath for 5 to 7 cm. (*E*) A new hiatus is opened approximately 30 mm above the old hiatus, and a large Penrose drain tube is passed through the new hiatus to stretch the bladder flat. The submucosal tunnel is constructed to a minimum of 15 mm in width and 30 mm in length toward the bladder neck. (*F*) The remodeled duplex ureter is then gently guided through the tunnel and anchored at a point 10 mm distal to the old hiatus where it is secured to the bladder. As a result, the total length of the submucosal tunnel is approximately 40 mm. A 6-Fr feeding tube is placed only in the upper pole ureter for temporary drainage during the first 4 days. A urethral catheter is left and is removed on postoperative day 7. (*From* Yamazaki, and colleagues[31])

presentation with fUTI. After a median follow-up of 6.1 years (range: 1–14.3 years), postoperative UTIs occurred in 15.6% (n = 5), and no patient underwent a secondary endoscopic procedure. Intermittent day wetting was observed in 6.3% (n = 2), which subsided in follow-up.[37]

Although as one-third of patients have historically undergone secondary procedures following lower tract reconstruction, it seems that few suffer from significant bladder dysfunction long-term and continence is excellent, even for those undergoing surgery for ectopic ureteroceles.

LOWER TRACT APPROACH: ENDOSCOPIC URETEROCELE INCISION/PUNCTURE

Endoscopic decompression of ureteroceles is perhaps the most widely performed approach,

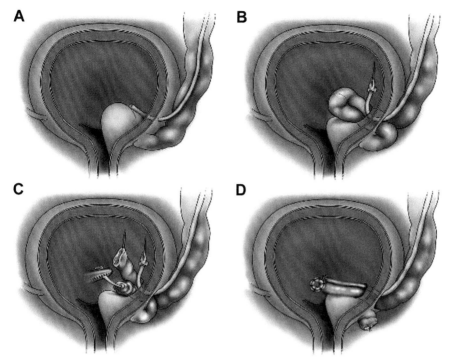

Fig. 6. The "In-and-Out" method of lower urinary tract reconstruction in young infants. (*A*) Mucosal incision is made along the lower edge of the orifice of the lower pole ureter. (*B*) A 7-0 polydioxanone suture is placed on the orifice of the lower pole ureter to facilitate the dissection. The lower pole ureter is dissected out and cut open. (*C*) The mucosal layer of the distal stump/ureterocele is detached as distally as possible and ligated intramurally. (*D*) Common sheath reimplantation is performed through a submucosal tunnel. (*From* Ting CS and Chang PY.[34])

Box 6
Operative techniques for endoscopic ureterocele puncture

- Diathermy
  - 3-Fr flexible monopolar "Bugbee" wire
  - Cutting current should be high enough to ensure a clean puncture.
- Holmium:Yag laser[42]
  - 30W laser with either 272 or 550 micron end-firing laser fiber with 10 to 18W power (0.5–0.8 J and 5–9 Hz) depending on subjective impression of thickness of ureterocele wall.
  - The fiber may be passed through a 4-Fr ureteral catheter for stability.
- The bladder should be incompletely filled to achieve maximal ureterocele distension for puncture/incision irrespective of the thermal energy used.
  - For intravesical ureteroceles, the puncture can be low on the front of the ureterocele, allowing collapsed tissue to establish an antireflux valve.[39]
  - For ectopic ureterocele, a single puncture of the intravesical portion of the ureterocele can be made just proximal to the bladder neck.[39]
  - Incising distally on the ureterocele, close to the bladder floor, may prevent de novo VUR.
  - Decompression of the ureterocele may be difficult to achieve if the Bugbee electrode displaces the inner mucosal coat of the ureterocele away from the outer layer.[39]
  - An alternate approach to single-puncture technique is the stented and unstented "watering-can" approach.
    - At least 2 punctures or up to 10 to 20 punctures are created to fenestrate the ureterocele wall, depending on the size of the ureterocele and perceived wall thickness.[48,59]

useful in any age patient and under any circumstance, especially during acute UTI. The procedure is summarized in **Box 6** and **Fig. 7**.

What is the incidence of iatrogenic VUR, and does it matter? De novo (or iatrogenic) VUR is the most common outcome following endoscopic treatment of ureteroceles, occurring in 22% to 100% of cases.[38,39] Sander and colleagues observed a lower incidence of de novo VUR among patients with SSU as compared with those with DSU (5/18 [27.8%] versus 18/32 [56.2%], *P* = .0773), which resulted in a lower incidence of secondary surgery as well (3.8% vs 73.7%, *P* < .0001).[40] In contrast, among 46 children with ectopic DSUs, Adorisio and colleagues found that

only 5 patients (10%) developed de novo VUR (grade 3 in 3 and grade 2 in 2), 3 of whom underwent endoscopic implantation of Deflux and 2 resolved spontaneously. Yin and Yang assessed the incidence of de novo VUR among 75 patients (12 [16%] men, 63 [84%] women) treated for unilateral ectopic DSUs treated by transurethral ureterocele incision (TUI) (29, 38.6%), transurethral ureterocele puncture (TUP) (10, 13.3%), UPPN (25, 33.3%), or common sheath ureteral reimplantation (CSR) (11, 14.6%).[41] Multivariate binary logistic regression analysis for adverse outcomes, in general, found a statistically significantly greater odds ratio for TUI and TUP as compared with UPPN (odds ratio [OR] = 11.049, *P* = .004 and OR 33.222, *P* = .002, respectively).[41]

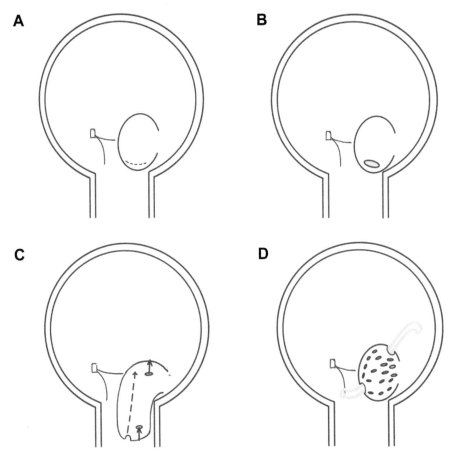

Fig. 7. Technique of incision or puncture of ureteroceles. (*A*) For an intravesical ureterocele a 3-Fr Bugbee electrode is used to extend the opening transversely, low on the anterior wall to preserve a flap of decompressed ureterocele. (*B*) Alternatively a single puncture low on the anterior wall creates a flap and results in lower likelihood of iatrogenic VUR. (*C*) For an ectopic ureterocele it is necessary to drain urethral segment without leaving occluding distal lip; this can be achieved by longitudinal incision extending from distal extent of ureterocele through the bladder neck sufficiently proximal to ensure that bladder neck closure does not occlude opening. Alternatively, by puncturing urethral and intravesical segments of ureterocele through and through, satisfactory drainage is achieved. (*D*) The "watering can" technique relies on multiple punctures, usually with Holmium laser to provide maximal drainage of the ureterocele; this may be combined with insertion of a ureteral stent. (*Adapted from* Blyth and colleagues *J Urol.* Mar 1993;149(3):556 to 9.)

Table 7
Outcomes following diathermy transurethral ureterocele incision versus Holmium:Yag laser transurethral ureterocele puncture

Variable		Holmium:Yag TUP	Diathermy TUI	P
Method		Holmium:Yag 30W laser with either 272 or 550 micron end-firing laser fiber with 10–18W power (0.5–0.8 J and 5–9 Hz) depending on subjective impression of thickness of ureterocele wall. The fiber was passed through a 4-Fr ureteral catheter for stability and 4–10 punctures were performed at the base of the bladder neck or trigone.	Incision at base of ureterocele, close to the bladder neck and trigonal wall with straight electrode through 10F pediatric cystoscope	
N (%)		64 (100)	26 (100)	-
Females		55 (85.9)	21 (80.7)	n.s.
DSU		53 (82.8)	22 (84.6)	n.s.
Median age at TUI/TUP, (range) months		6.3 (1–168)	5.9 (1–123)	n.s.
Presentation				
Prenatal hydro		43 (67.2)	15 (57.5)	n.s.
fUTI		15 (21.9)	8 (30.8)	<0.05
Screening US		6 (10.9)	2 (7.7)	n.s.
Orthotopic		15 (23)	5 (19.2)	n.s
Ectopic		49 (77)	21 (80.7)	n.s.
No. of Treatments Performed				
1	Total	59 (92)	24 (92.3)	n.s.
	Orthotopic	14 (93.3)	5 (100)	n.s.
	Ectopic	45 (76.3)	19 (79.2)	n.s
2	Total	5 (8)	2 97.7)	n.s
	Orthotopic	0 (0)	0 (0)	n.s.
	Ectopic	5 (100)	2 (100)	n.s.
Outcomes				
fUTI		15 (23.4)	10 (38.5)	<0.05
De novo	Orthotopic	2 (25)	5 (31.3)	<0.05
VUR	Ectopic	6 (750	11 (68.7)	<0.05
Reimplantation		7 (10.9)	9 (34.6)	<0.05
UPPN		5 (7.8)	4 (15.4)	<0.05

Abbreviations: n.s., nonsignificant; US, ultrasound.
Adapted from Caione and colleagues *Front Pediatr.* 2019;7:106.

Byun and Merguerian investigated the effect of ureterocele location (ectopic vs orthotopic, 12 studies, 431 patients), anatomy (SSU vs DSU, 5 studies, 177 patients), and presence of VUR preoperatively (7 studies, 255 patients) on reoperation rates following TUI/TUP.[13] Although endoscopic management is effective in decompressing the affected moiety, iatrogenic VUR is a likely outcome.

Reoperation rates following TUI/TUP seem to be driven mostly by the presence of VUR rather than persistence of hydronephrosis and are more likely seen in ectopic DSUs rather than intravesical SSUs.[13] Subgroup analysis "implies that ureterocele location and renal anatomy, and preoperative vesicoureteral reflux are proxies for trigonal distortion, rather than independent risk factors with

Table 8
Cox proportional hazard model identified risk factors for febrile urinary tract infection following transurethral ureterocele incision

Variable	Risk Ratio	95% CI	P
Female	11.6	2.213–214.0	<0.01
DSU	7.61	1.451–140.0	0.01
Unchanged hydronephrosis	65.0	7.949–1340	<0.01
Ectopic ureterocele	4.36	1.120–28.69	0.03

Adapted from Moriya and colleagues BJU Int. Sep 2017;120(3):409 to 415.

an additive effect on reoperation."[13] Revisiting Smith's editorial, though, surgeon bias toward correction of reflux in duplex systems or iatrogenic reflux may be the impetus behind secondary surgery, rather than symptoms.

VUR following endoscopic treatment may occur following endoscopic puncture, particularly into

larger ureteroceles with poor muscular backing. In these circumstances, a traditional approach relies on transvesical excision of the ureterocele, reconstruction of the floor of the bladder, and ureteral reimplantation. However, a nonsurgical approach—relying on antimicrobial prophylaxis—may result in resolution or downgrading of VUR severity while avoiding recurrent UTI.

Does the method of ureterocele decompression (TUI vs TUP) influence the incidence of de novo VUR? Caione and colleagues compared outcomes of traditional diathermy TUI (n = 26) against laser TUP (n = 64)[42] (**Table 7**). Overall, endoscopic management resulted in decompression of 92% of orthotopic and ectopic ureteroceles treated, neither TUI or TUP demonstrating an advantage for resolution of hydronephrosis. In general, orthotopic ureteroceles had better outcomes than ectopic ureteroceles.[42] However, TUP outperformed TUI in the incidence of fUTIs (23.4% vs 38.5%, $P < .05$), de novo VUR mostly into the upper pole (29.7% vs 61.5%, $P < .05$), and further open surgery (18% vs 50%, $P < .05$).[42] Because de novo VUR was only sought in patients with

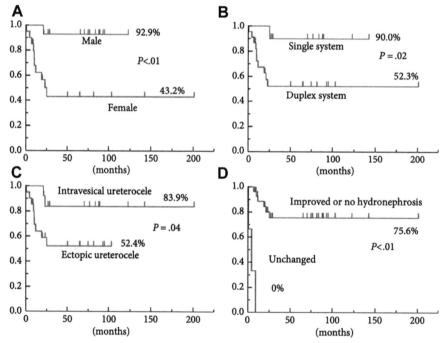

Fig. 8. Symptomatic UTI-free rate after endoscopic incision based on each risk factor. (*A*) Male versus female. The symptomatic UTI-free rate after endoscopic incision (EI) was 92.9% in boys and 43.2% in girls ($P < .01$). (*B*) Single-system versus duplex system ureterocele. The symptomatic UTI-free rate after EI was 90.0% in patients with a single-system and 52.3% in those with a duplex system ureterocele ($P = .02$). (*C*) Intravesical ureterocele versus ectopic ureterocele. The symptomatic UTI-free rate after EI was 83.9% in patients with an intravesical ureterocele and 52.4% in patients with an ectopic ureterocele ($P = .04$). (*D*) Improved or no hydronephrosis versus unchanged hydronephrosis on postoperative ultrasonography. The symptomatic UTI-free rate after EI was 75.6% in patients with improved or no hydronephrosis and 0% with unchanged hydronephrosis ($P < .01$). (*From* Moriya and colleagues *BJU Int.* Sep 2017;120(3):409 to 415.)

persistent hydronephrosis and fUTI, the true incidence of iatrogenic VUR in this population cannot be known. Yet, these data suggest that clinically significant de novo VUR afflicts few patients following endoscopic treatment, but fUTI is frequently coexisting and may drive more extensive surgery.

If recurrent fUTIs, progressive hydronephrosis, and bladder outlet obstruction (BOO) are the strictest indications for secondary surgery, what is the incidence of each? Moriya and colleagues investigated the prevalence of risk factors associated with symptomatic UTI among 36 children with DSUs (n = 23) and SSUs (n = 13) treated by TUI.[43] The symptomatic UTI-free rate after TUI was 65.6%, 11 children having 1 to 2 UTIs less than 25 months after TUI. The Cox-proportional hazard model identified female sex, DSU, ectopic position, and unchanged hydronephrosis as significant risk factors for the development of post-TUI fUTIs—findings that corroborate earlier studies[13,40,43–46] (**Table 8**, **Fig. 8**). Because VUR was not found to increase the risk for fUTI, the authors inferred—with justification—that a nonoperative approach should be initially considered. Not unlike isolated primary VUR, most VUR following TUI do not require surgery.

TUP/TUI resolves obstructive hydronephrosis with decompression rates ranging from 78% to 97%.[40,43,47,48] Chowdhary and colleagues reported on 43 patients treated over 10 years for 17 ectopic (8 DSUs, 5 SSUs) and 22 orthotopic (14 DSUs, 8 SSUs) ureteroceles (see **Table 8**). Among patients with ectopic ureteroceles, hydronephrosis improved in 61% (8/13) and remained stable in 38.5% (5/13), but no patient underwent second decompression to treat hydronephrosis nor suffered from incontinence or BOO. Recurrent fUTIs did occur in 2 of these children who ultimately underwent UPPN (n = 1) and CSR (n = 1). Eighty-six percent (18/21) of children with orthotopic ureterocele were successfully treated with TUI alone. Four patients were managed entirely nonoperatively. Four children underwent open surgery as an initial approach, all of whom had fUTI as well as BOO (n = 1), and CRF (n = 1).

CLINICS CARE POINTS

- At best, upper pole moieties of duplex systems associated with ureteroceles provide 16% of total renal function.
- Non-operative management should be considered for (a) good functioning upper poles with no evidence of high grade obstruction or (b) non-functioning upper poles consistent with cystic dysplastic moieties.
- The risk of open conversion, urinoma/leak, stimp infection and renal loss during UPPN is similar for laparoscopic intraperitoneal, laparascopic retroperitoneal, robotic intraperitoneal and robotic retroperitoneal; no technique proving statistically significantly advantageous. In limited series, robotic approaches may be associated with a lower risk for renal function loss.
- Performing UU when there is significant size disparity between the upper and lower pole ureter may result in stump infection in up to 12% of patients when performed high. For that reason, it is preferable to perform low UU.
- Standard excision of the ureterocele with re-implantation carries up to 35% risk for persistent reflux for which secondary endoscopy or open procedures may be required.
- Contemporary studies on patients managed endoscopically have called into question the clinical significance of post incision/puncture vesicoureteral reflux.

SUPPLEMENTARY DATA

Supplementary data related to this article can be found online at https://doi.org/10.1016/j.thorsurg.2023.04.015.

REFERENCES

1. Timberlake MD, Corbett ST. Minimally invasive techniques for management of the ureterocele and ectopic ureter: upper tract versus lower tract approach. Urol Clin North Am 2015;42(1):61–76.
2. Kroovand RL. Ureterocele. Urol Clin North Am 1983;10(3):445–9.
3. Reitelman C, Perlmutter AD. Management of obstructing ectopic ureteroceles. Urol Clin North Am 1990;17(2):317–28.
4. Chwalla R. The process of formation of cystic dilation of the vesical end of the ureter and of diverticula at the ureteral ostium. Urol Cutan Rev 1927;31(499).
5. Stephens FD, Smith ED and Hutson J, Ureteroceles on duplex ureters, In: Stephens FD, Smith ED and Hutson J., *Congenital Anomalies of the kidney, urinary and genital tracts*, 2nd ed., 2002, London, UK. Martin Dunetz, 243–262, chap 24.
6. Stephens D. Caecoureteroceles and Concepts on the Embryology and Aetiology of Ureteroceles. ANZ J Surg 1971;40(3):239–48.
7. Subbiah N, Stephens D. Stenotic ureterocele. Aust N Z J Surg 1972;41(3):257–63.

8. Brock WA, Kaplan GW. Ectopic ureteroceles in children. J Urol 1978;119(6):800–3.

9. Mandell J, Colodny AH, Lebowitz R, et al. Ureteroceles in infants and children. J Urol 1980;123(6):921–6.

10. Uson AC, Lattimer JK, Melicow MM. Ureteroceles in infants and children: a report based on 44 cases. Pediatrics 1961;27:971–83.

11. Decter RM, Roth DR, Gonzales ET. Individualized treatment of ureteroceles. J Urol 1989;142(2 Pt 2):535–7 [discussion 542-3.

12. Sen S, Beasley SW, Ahmed S, et al. Renal function and vesicoureteric reflux in children with ureteroceles. Pediatr Surg Int 1992;7:192–4.

13. Byun E, Merguerian PA. A meta-analysis of surgical practice patterns in the endoscopic management of ureteroceles. J Urol 2006;176(4 Pt 2):1871–7 [discussion: 1877].

14. Vates TS, Bukowski T, Triest J, et al. Is there a best alternative to treating the obstructed upper pole? J Urol 1996;156(2 Pt 2):744–6.

15. Merlini E, Lelli Chiesa P. Obstructive ureterocele-an ongoing challenge. World J Urol 2004;22(2):107–14.

16. Han MY, Gibbons MD, Belman AB, et al. Indications for nonoperative management of ureteroceles. J Urol 2005;174(4 Pt 2):1652–5 [discussion: 1655-6].

17. Arena F, Nicotina A, Cruccetti A, et al. Can histologic changes of the upper pole justify a conservative approach in neonatal duplex ectopic ureterocele? Pediatr Surg Int 2002;18(8):681–4.

18. Maruo K, Nishinaka K. Conservative treatment of asymptomatic ectopic ureterocele: A report of two cases. IJU Case Rep 2020;3(2):40–3.

19. Shankar KR, Vishwanath N, Rickwood AM. Outcome of patients with prenatally detected duplex system ureterocele; natural history of those managed expectantly. J Urol 2001;165(4):1226–8.

20. Direnna T, Leonard MP. Watchful waiting for prenatally detected ureteroceles. J Urol 2006;175(4):1493–5 [discussion: 1495].

21. You D, Bang JK, Shim M, et al. Analysis of the late outcome of laparoscopic heminephrectomy in children with duplex kidneys. BJU Int 2010;106(2):250–4.

22. Neheman A, Kord E, Strine AC, et al. Pediatric Partial Nephrectomy for Upper Urinary Tract Duplication Anomalies: A Comparison Between Different Surgical Approaches and Techniques. Urology 2019;125:196–201.

23. Joyeux L, Lacreuse I, Schneider A, et al. Long-term functional renal outcomes after retroperitoneoscopic upper pole heminephrectomy for duplex kidney in children: a multicenter cohort study. Surg Endosc 2017;31(3):1241–9.

24. Esposito C, Escolino M, Miyano G, et al. A comparison between laparoscopic and retroperitoneoscopic approach for partial nephrectomy in children with duplex kidney: a multicentric survey. World J Urol 2016;34(7):939–48.

25. Luo J, Tan XH, Liu X, et al. Anatomy and management of upper moiety vascular variation in children with duplex kidney. J Pediatr Surg 2019;54(10):2130–3.

26. Romao RL, Figueroa V, Salle JL, et al. Laparoscopic ureteral ligation (clipping): a novel, simple procedure for pediatric urinary incontinence due to ectopic ureters associated with non-functioning upper pole renal moieties. J Pediatr Urol 2014;10(6):1089–94.

27. Lopes RI, Fernandez N, Koyle MA, et al. Clinical Outcomes of the Upper Urinary Tract after Ureteral Clipping for Treatment of Low Functioning or Nonfunctioning Renal Moieties. J Urol 2018;199(2):558–64.

28. Li Z, Psooy K, Morris M, et al. Laparoscopic ligation of ectopic ureter in pediatric patients: a safe surgical option for the management of urinary incontinence due to ectopic ureters. Pediatr Surg Int 2021;37(5):667–71.

29. Chacko JK, Koyle MA, Mingin GC, et al. Ipsilateral ureteroureterostomy in the surgical management of the severely dilated ureter in ureteral duplication. J Urol 2007;178(4 Pt 2):1689–92.

30. McLeod DJ, Alpert SA, Ural Z, et al. Ureteroureterostomy irrespective of ureteral size or upper pole function: a single center experience. J Pediatr Urol 2014;10(4):616–9.

31. Kawal T, Srinivasan AK, Talwar R, et al. Ipsilateral ureteroureterostomy: does function of the obstructed moiety matter? J Pediatr Urol 2019;15(1):50.e1–6.

32. Biles MJ, Finkelstein JB, Silva MV, et al. Innovation in Robotics and Pediatric Urology: Robotic Ureteroureterostomy for Duplex Systems with Ureteral Ectopia. J Endourol 2016;30(10):1041–8.

33. Lee YS, Hah YS, Kim MJ, et al. Factors associated with complications of the ureteral stump after proximal ureteroureterostomy. J Urol 2012;188(5):1890–4.

34. Yamazaki Y, Setoguchi K, Yago R, et al. Common sheath reimplantation with ureteral plication: a useful technique for the management of ectopic ureterocele. Int J Urol 1999;6(10):532–5.

35. de Jong TP, Dik P, Klijn AJ, et al. Ectopic ureterocele: results of open surgical therapy in 40 patients. J Urol 2000;164(6):2040–3 [discussion: 2043-4].

36. Beganović A, Klijn AJ, Dik P, et al. Ectopic ureterocele: long-term results of open surgical therapy in 54 patients. J Urol 2007;178(1):251–4.

37. Ting CS, Chang PY. An alternative lower tract approach to ectopic duplex system ureteroceles feasible in young children. J Pediatr Urol 2023;19(1):87.e1–6.

38. Coplen DE, Duckett JW. The modern approach to ureteroceles. J Urol 1995;153(1):166–71.

39. Hagg MJ, Mourachov PV, Snyder HM, et al. The modern endoscopic approach to ureterocele. J Urol 2000;163(3):940–3.

40. Sander JC, Bilgutay AN, Stanasel I, et al. Outcomes of endoscopic incision for the treatment of uterocele in children at a single institution. J Urol 2015; 193(2):662–6.

41. Yin X, Yang Y. Risk factors for postoperative adverse outcomes and secondary surgery in pediatric patients with unilateral ectopic ureterocele associated with the duplex system. J Pediatr Urol 2022. https://doi.org/10.1016/j.jpurol.2022.10.022.

42. Caione P, Gerocarni Nappo S, Collura G, et al. Minimally Invasive Laser Treatment of Ureterocele. Front Pediatr 2019;7:106.

43. Moriya K, Nakamura M, Nishimura Y, et al. Prevalence of and risk factors for symptomatic urinary tract infection after endoscopic incision for the treatment of ureterocele in children. BJU Int 2017;120(3): 409–15.

44. Di Renzo D, Ellsworth PI, Caldamone AA, et al. Transurethral puncture for ureterocele-which factors dictate outcomes? J Urol 2010;184(4 Suppl): 1620–4.

45. Castagnetti M, Cimador M, Sergio M, et al. Transurethral incision of duplex system ureteroceles in neonates: does it increase the need for secondary surgery in intravesical and ectopic cases? BJU Int 2004;93(9):1313–7.

46. Cooper CS, Passerini-Glazel G, Hutcheson JC, et al. Long-term followup of endoscopic incision of ureteroceles: intravesical versus extravesical. J Urol 2000; 164(3 Pt 2):1097–9 [discussion: 1099-100].

47. Adorisio O, Elia A, Landi L, et al. Effectiveness of primary endoscopic incision in treatment of ectopic ureterocele associated with duplex system. Urology 2011;77(1):191–4.

48. Palmer BW, Greger H, Mannas DB, et al. Comparison of endoscopic ureterocele decompression techniques. Preliminary experience–is the watering can puncture superior? J Urol 2011;186(4 Suppl):1700–3.

49. Abedinzadeh M, Nouralizadeh A, Radfar MH, et al. Transperitoneal laparoscopic heminephrectomy in duplex kidneys: a one centre experience. Ger Med Sci 2012;10:Doc05.

50. Cabezali D, Maruszewski P, López F, et al. Complications and late outcome in transperitoneal laparoscopic heminephrectomy for duplex kidney in children. J Endourol 2013;27(2):133–8.

51. Dingemann C, Petersen C, Kuebler JF, et al. Laparoscopic transperitoneal heminephrectomy for duplex kidney in infants and children: a comparative study. J Laparoendosc Adv Surg Tech 2013;23(10):889–93.

52. Golebiewski A, Losin M, Murawski M, et al. Laparoscopic versus open upper pole heminephroureterectomy for the treatment of duplex kidneys in children. J Laparoendosc Adv Surg Tech 2013; 23(11):942–5.

53. Marte A, Papparella A, Pintozzi L. Laparoscopic upper pole heminephroureterectomy in children: Seven-year experience. Afr J Paediatr Surg 2015; 12(4):227–31.

54. Szklarz MT, Ruiz J, Moldes JM, et al. Laparoscopic Upper-pole Heminephrectomy for the Management of Duplex Kidney: Outcomes of a Multicenter Cohort. Urology 2021;156:245–50.

55. Chen Z, Tang ZY, Fan BY, et al. Retroperitoneoscopic upper pole nephroureterectomy in duplex kidney: focus on the role of dilated upper pole ureter. Urol J 2014;10(4):1046–53.

56. MacDonald C, Small R, Flett M, et al. Predictors of complications following retroperitoneoscopic total and partial nephrectomy. J Pediatr Surg 2019; 54(2):331–4.

57. Wadham B, DeSilva A, Connolly T, et al. The place of retroperitoneoscopic hemi-nephroureterectomy for duplex kidney in children; risk of damage to the remnant moiety and strategies to reduce the risk. J Pediatr Urol 2021;17(5):708.e1–8.

58. Roshan A, MacNeily AE. Dorsal lumbotomy for pediatric upper pole hemi-nephrectomy: Back (door) to the future? J Pediatr Urol 2020;16(4):480.e1–7.

59. Kajbafzadeh A, Salmasi AH, Payabvash S, et al. Evolution of endoscopic management of ectopic ureterocele: a new approach. J Urol 2007;177(3): 1118–23 [discussion: 1123].

Vesicoureteral Reflux
Current Care Trends and Future Possibilities

Eric M. Bortnick, MD, Caleb P. Nelson, MD, MPH*

KEYWORDS

- Vesicoureteral reflux • Urinary tract infection • Continuous antibiotic prophylaxis
- Ureteral reimplantation • Predictive models • Machine learning

KEY POINTS

- Investigations over the past 2 decades have improved our understanding of the natural history of vesicoureteral reflux (VUR) and helped identify those at higher risk of both VUR itself as well as its potential severe sequelae.
- Although continuous antibiotic prophylaxis (CAP) has been demonstrated to be effective in reducing the risk of recurrent urinary tract infection (UTI) in children with VUR, efforts continue to identify those children most likely to benefit from CAP and to minimize adverse consequences.
- VUR is associated with progressive renal injury and scarring, particularly in the context of febrile UTI; multiple recurrent infections, delay in initiating treatment, and deferred diagnosis of VUR are associated with higher risk of renal scarring in young children.
- Advanced analytic tools including artificial intelligence and machine learning have shown promise in distilling large volumes of granular data into practical tools that clinicians can use to guide diagnosis and management decisions for their patients and to identify specific patient most likely to benefit from diagnosis.
- Surgical treatment, when indicated, remains highly effective and is associated with low morbidity.

EPIDEMIOLOGY AND NATURAL HISTORY OF VESICOURETERAL REFLUX

Vesicoureteral reflux (VUR) is the retrograde flow of urine from the bladder to the upper urinary tract. VUR is associated with increased risk of urinary tract infections (UTIs), pyelonephritis, and upper tract damage such as renal scar formation leading to decreased renal function. "Primary VUR" is caused by immaturity or structural abnormality of the ureterovesical junction, resulting in failure of the normal antireflux mechanism; the bladder and ureter are otherwise anatomically and neurologically normal. "Secondary VUR" is reflux that occurs in the setting of an abnormal lower urinary tract, such as in bladder exstrophy, posterior urethral valves, or neurogenic bladder associated with spina bifida. In this paper the authors focus primarily on primary VUR. VUR is commonly diagnosed by voiding cystourethrogram and is graded on a 5-level scale initially proposed by the International Reflux Study Committee,[1] based on height of reflux in the upper tract and degree of dilation. Radionuclide cystogram (RNC) is an alternative to voiding cystourethrography (VCUG) and continues to be used at selected centers; advantages include low radiation exposure and continuous imaging (which may increase sensitivity), but anatomic detail is limited, and specialized equipment and radioisotopes are required.

The true population prevalence of VUR is not known, as the studies required to determine this accurately would be unethical. However, limited older data suggest that overall 1% to 2% of infants have VUR.[2] It is clear however that VUR is much

Department of Pediatric Urology, Boston Children's Hospital, 300 Longwood Avenue, Boston, MA 02115, USA
* Corresponding author.
E-mail address: Caleb.nelson@childrens.harvard.edu

Urol Clin N Am 50 (2023) 391–402
https://doi.org/10.1016/j.ucl.2023.04.003
0094-0143/23/© 2023 Elsevier Inc. All rights reserved.

more prevalent among certain groups, including children with history of urinary tract dilation (UTD), febrile UTI, and family history of VUR. Gender is also associated with prevalence of VUR, with more boys diagnosed with VUR during infancy, whereas among older children, girls are more likely to be found to have VUR (primarily associated with UTI). The gender difference in prevalence is likely driven largely by the increased prevalence of UTD prenatally among boys, resulting in more frequent testing of infant boys as part of the workup for UTD, as well as the susceptibility of infant boys (particularly if uncircumcised) to febrile UTI; among older children, both febrile UTI and VUR are more common in girls.[3,4] For example, girls comprised 80% of patients enrolled in the International Reflux Study[5] and 92% of subjects in the RIVUR trial.[6] A recent review of infants with VUR up to age 24 months supports the earlier reports, with male:female ratio of 3:1 from 0 to 6 months old and roughly 1:1 from 21 to 24 month old.[7]

Although historically VUR has been stated to be less prevalent in nonwhite children, and particularly uncommon in children of African descent,[4] recent widespread conversations have questioned the use of race as a risk factor, arguing that race is primarily a social construct and thus a proxy for other factors that should be used for risk prediction.[8] The true relationship of race (whatever that is thought to mean) with VUR requires further research to fully elucidate.

It has long been recognized that VUR resolves spontaneously in a large proportion of children. Lower grades of VUR are more likely to resolve, which has been the premise on which surveillance (with or without antimicrobial prophylaxis) is based. The ability to predict which patients with VUR will resolve would have profound management implications, and efforts to develop more accurate predictive models go back many years. Estrada and colleagues used a database of more than 2000 patients to identify factors associated with spontaneous resolution, including VUR grade, age at diagnosis, gender, laterality, reason for diagnosis (UTI vs UTD), and duplication anomalies, and developed a calculator to provide individual probability of resolution.[9] This calculator provides resolution probability over 1 to 5 years from diagnosis. More recently, Kirsch and colleagues introduced the VUR Index as a predictive model of VUR improvement and resolution in children younger than 2 years with newly diagnosed reflux.[10] Based on 229 patients, this model includes gender, VUR timing on VCUG, presence of ureteral anomalies, and high-grade reflux. VUR improvement/resolution rates over 2 years was 89%, 69%, 53%, 16%, and 11% for VUR Index scores of 1 to 5 to 6, respectively.[10] The same group later validated the VUR Index as prognostic for VUR resolution in a multiinstitutional study in 369 patients younger than 2 years and also showed the validity of VUR Index for reflux resolution in children older than 2 years in a multiinstitutional series of 261 patients.[11,12]

Another metric proposed to be associated with VUR resolution is the ureteral diameter ratio (UDR). This is the ratio of distal ureteral diameter to the L1-L3 vertebral distance as measured on VCUG. Cooper and colleagues first reported that the mean UDR of those that underwent surgical correction (n = 42) was significantly greater than those whose reflux resolved (n = 37) and that on logistic regression analysis UDR was significantly associated with VUR outcome.[13] A 2017 external validation of UDR in 147 patients found that although reflux grade and UDR were predictive of reflux resolution on a multivariate model, UDR had a higher likelihood ratio and was more predictive of reflux resolution than grade alone. In addition, they found there seemed to be a specified UDR cutoff of 0.43 in which no patients achieved early spontaneous resolution, which differs from standard reflux grading in which resolution may be achieved at any grade when considering other factors.[14]

Thus, predicting spontaneous resolution of VUR remains a rather speculative endeavor, but several models exist that can help provide guidance for clinical decision-making.

DIAGNOSIS OF VESICOURETERAL REFLUX IN THE CONTEXT OF URINARY TRACT DILATION

UTD is one of the most common congenital anomalies diagnosed on prenatal screening, and UTD has long been noted to be associated with VUR, and therefore postnatal VCUG has commonly been recommended as part of the newborn workup for many infants with UTD.[15] Despite this, the ability to delineate which patients with UTD will have significant pathology from those that do not has been challenging for researchers and clinicians. A variety of scoring systems have been proposed seeking to risk stratify infants with UTD, most recently the "UTD" consensus classification system.[16] However, it is clear that ultrasound is not good at distinguishing those with and without VUR. Although studies have shown that VUR is more common in patients with UTD compared with those without UTD,[17,18] there is little correlation between degree of UTD and risk of VUR (ie, prevalence of VUR is roughly equivalent, around 15%, for each category of UTD).[17]

Similarly, another study of almost 500 patients with prenatal UTD found that, among those who had a VCUG performed, the prevalence of any VUR and higher-grade VUR (defined as VUR grade > II) was not significantly different between UTD classification groups (P0, P1, P2, P3).[19] These findings are consistent with prior studies that used different classification systems for UTD, which also found no correlation between renal dilation severity and risk for VUR.[20-22]

So which infants with UTD should undergo neonatal VCUG to assess for VUR? The UTD consensus panel recommended that infants with grade UTD P3 should undergo a VCUG, whereas evaluation with VCUG in infants with grade UTD P1 and P2 was left "to the discretion of the clinician."[16] However, it has been pointed out that, because there is little evidence that VUR is significantly more common among infants with higher grades of UTD, VCUG should be performed based not primarily on UTD grade but on presence of specific ultrasound findings that suggest higher likelihood of high-grade VUR, such as ureteral dilation, or findings suggestive of lower urinary tract obstruction, such as bladder abnormalities.[23]

DIAGNOSIS OF VESICOURETERAL REFLUX IN THE CONTEXT OF FEBRILE URINARY TRACT INFECTION

As VUR is frequently identified on VCUG as part of the workup after a child has a febrile UTI, changes in guidelines for management of UTI in children have affected diagnosis and treatment of VUR. The American Academy of Pediatrics (AAP) guidelines for workup after febrile UTI in young children have shifted over time. In 1999, the guidelines recommended a renal and bladder ultrasound (RBUS) and VCUG in children age 2 months to 2 years who developed febrile UTI.[24] New guidelines released in 2011 dropped the VCUG recommendation and stated that VCUG should only be performed if the RBUS was abnormal or if the child developed a second febrile UTI.[25] Other guidelines, such as those from the UK National Institute for Health and Clinical Excellence (NICE) in 2007, also recommended against VCUG after initial febrile UTI.[26] There has been debate regarding the recommendations to defer VCUG, with organizations such as the Section on Urology of the AAP pushing back against this change.[27]

One premise of the revised guidelines is that RBUS, which is still recommended after the initial UTI, is a useful screening test for VUR and other conditions associated with UTI. This implication is demonstrated by the recommendation that after first febrile UTI, VCUG should only be performed if the RBUS is abnormal. This raises the question of how accurate RBUS is as a screening test for VCUG-demonstrated conditions such as VUR. Evidence suggests that RBUS is in fact not particularly sensitive or specific for VUR, and a negative RBUS does not rule out VUR[28]; such findings argue for both RBUS and VCUG to be performed. On the other hand, other investigators have made the argument that even the RBUS is unnecessary after the first febrile UTI based on cost-effectiveness calculations.[29] Alternatively, another study found that limiting RBUS after febrile UTI to children with non-*Escherichia coli* infection or recurrent UTI detected all patients with high-grade VUR while reducing the number of normal RBUS performed.[30] These positions remain outside the mainstream however, and most guidelines and experts continue to recommend at least an RBUS after initial febrile UTI in every child.[31]

The result of the shifting guidelines over the past 20 years has been significant drop in the frequency of evaluation with VCUG after febrile UTI in young children.[32-34] There is still variability, however, and there is also evidence that adherence to the 2011 AAP guidelines varies by specialty.[34,35]

Given the changes in practice patterns, research efforts have shifted to assessment of the potential consequences of deferred VCUG (and therefore deferred VUR diagnosis) on infectious and renal outcomes. One might expect that greater selectivity in VCUG utilization (limited to those with abnormal RBUS or recurrent febrile UTI) would increase the yield of these studies, with increases in VUR prevalence and severity. However, one might also be concerned that the delay in evaluation could result in more children developing renal scarring due to recurrent pyelonephritis if their VUR diagnosis is delayed. To look at this, Lee and colleagues compared children presenting with febrile UTI in 2005 versus those in 2015 to determine whether the changes in guidelines over time was associated with different clinical presentation and renal outcomes. As expected, those diagnosed in 2015 had higher likelihood of recurrent UTI (odds ratio [OR] 3.01, 95% confidence interval [CI] 2.18–4.16, $P < .0001$), and although the proportion with VUR did not vary by time period (OR 0.98, 95% CI 0.77–1.23, $P = .85$), renal scarring was more common in 2015 (OR 2.9, 95% CI 1.03–8.20, $P = .04$).[36] This raises the possibility that more children are developing acquired renal scarring before their initial VUR diagnosis; whether this scarring could have been prevented with earlier diagnosis is a critical question.

The relevance of such findings is complimented by the growing evidence of the association of febrile UTI and presence of VUR (particularly high-grade VUR) with renal scarring.[37] Yilmaz and colleagues compared children with nonfebrile UTI, first febrile UTI, and recurrent UTI and found that the highest incidence of both VUR and renal scarring in the group with recurrent UTI.[38] Another large analysis of prospective clinical trial data showed that the odds of renal scarring among those with recurrent UTI were more than 10 times higher than after a single febrile infection (OR 11.8, 95% CI: 4.1–34.4).[39] Children with febrile UTI in whom VUR is diagnosed later in childhood also tend to have high incidence of renal damage and scarring.[40,41] Clearly, having multiple febrile UTIs is potentially damaging to renal tissue. There is also evidence that delay of treatment of febrile UTI is associated with renal scarring, with longer delays resulting in higher likelihood of scarring on subsequent DMSA scan.[42] These findings reinforce the need for prompt evaluation and treatment of young children known to be at risk for UTI, such as those with VUR.

These data raise concerns about the deferral of VCUG and VUR diagnosis, but it is also likely that VCUG is indeed unnecessary in many children who have had a febrile UTI. Can we be more selective in whom VCUG is performed? In other words, instead of simply waiting for the second febrile UTI, can we identify those at highest risk for recurrent UTI and/or VUR and perform VCUG after the initial febrile UTI in just this group? Several groups have sought to identify factors that would facilitate such selectivity. A large Italian study found that non-E coli initial febrile UTI was associated with much higher risk of VUR (OR 2.74, 95% CI: 1.39–5.41, $P = 0.003$).[43] Other investigators have sought to use multivariable models to predict which children are most likely to have VUR on a VCUG. For example, a study from Japan found that non-E coli UTI (as well as other ultrasound findings, positive blood culture, and "poor clinical appearance") was associated with higher risk of high-grade (grade IV–V) VUR.[44] Roesch and colleagues developed a predictive model for VUR that included DMSA findings, duplex system, age, fever duration, number of febrile UTI's, and ultrasound findings to identify higher-risk patients, resulting in an area under the curve (AUC) of 0.686.[45] Breinbjerg and colleagues conducted a similar study and found that non-E coli UTI, abnormal RBUS, elevated creatinine, and delayed response to treatment (>48 h) were risk factors for grade III to V VUR (and abnormal DMSA).[46] Still another group reported that risk factors for high-grade VUR were recurrent UTI ($P < .001$), non-E coli pathogen ($P = .011$), and

abnormal RBUS[47]; various combinations of factors improved specificity but decreased sensitivity. Such models are potentially promising, but often are hindered by low numbers of patients and the intrinsic limitations of conventional multivariate regression analysis to incorporate large numbers of potential predictors. They also may require data elements that are not straightforward to obtain, as in the DMSA findings in the Roesch and colleagues' study.[45]

Another approach taken recently by certain investigators is to use advanced analytic techniques including machine learning and artificial intelligence to model relevant outcomes and predict which patients might benefit from certain interventions. For example, a group from the Massachusetts Institute of Technology and Boston Children's Hospital used a machine learning algorithm to study a large dataset of children with initial UTI, seeking to identify those most likely to have both VUR and recurrent UTI[48]; if such children could be reliably identified, VCUG could be limited just to these children after the initial febrile UTI. The algorithm performed with AUC of 0.76, using readily available variables. With further refinement, these advanced analytic tools are likely to dramatically affect our ability to "personalize" the post-UTI workup in children, limiting VCUG to those most likely to have VUR that will be associated with UTI recurrence (the group at highest risk of developing renal scarring).

DIAGNOSIS OF VESICOURETERAL REFLUX IN THE CONTEXT OF SIBLING SCREENING

It has long been recognized that VUR is common among relatives of VUR patients, and this has prompted screening of asymptomatic relatives (particularly siblings) for VUR in the past.[49] However, the evidence supporting sibling screening has been very limited. The 2010 American Urologic Association guidelines (updated 2017) cited the lack of evidence in not recommending systematic screening of siblings.[50] There is reason to believe that sibling screening for VUR is not cost-effective, and large numbers of siblings would need to be screened to prevent even a single UTI.[51] Analysis of claims data from a regional insurer showed that, although UTI incidence among siblings was significant (8.4%–10.4%), there was no difference in UTI incidence between screened and unscreened siblings, suggesting that screening may not reduce UTI risk among siblings.[52] More practically, there are many payers that will not reimburse for VCUG or RNC performed for the indication of sibling or other family history of VUR.

New Modalities for Vesicoureteral Reflux Diagnosis

VCUG has long been considered the gold standard for VUR diagnosis, but alternatives do exist.

Sonographic voiding urography using ultrasound contrast agents (sometimes termed a "voiding urosonogram") has been developed over the past decade. This technology uses the echogenic properties of gas-filled microspheres, which are instilled into the bladder via a catheter and then can be observed with ultrasound.[53,54] Paltiel and colleagues found that detection of VUR with this modality is comparable with that observed with VCUG,[55] and it has been argued that this technology is now mature enough that it could replace fluoroscopic VCUG.[56] The technology has the advantage of avoiding ionizing radiation and allows for prolonged imaging over multiple cycles. However, ongoing challenges include lack of standardization of grading, debatable ability to detect bladder or urethral anomalies, imaging limited to one side at a time, and substantial interoperator variability compounded by lack of trained technologists and radiologists with the technical skills to perform this imaging procedure.

TREATMENT OF VESICOURETERAL REFLUX: ANTIBIOTIC PROPHYLAXIS

Continuous antimicrobial prophylaxis (CAP) has been used since the 1970s,[57] based on the premise that if recurrent UTI can be prevented until the child's VUR resolves, antireflux surgery might be avoided. However, there has long been debate about whether CAP is actually effective in children with VUR. As noted previously, one of the arguments against early diagnosis of VUR is that CAP is not effective in preventing UTI recurrence. After all, if medical therapy is ineffective (and as only a small proportion of children with VUR will ever need surgery), there would be less benefit in diagnosing VUR. At the time that the 2011 AAP guidelines were released, a reasonable case could be made that the data supported this position, as several trials of CAP in the setting of VUR had produced equivocal results. However, many of these studies had significant limitations, and in 2014 the RIVUR study results were published. This study was the largest, most rigorously designed trial to date investigating the effect of CAP on UTI recurrence in children with VUR and showed that CAP reduced the risk of recurrent UTI by roughly half.[6] Subsequent meta-analyses have found that the preponderance of evidence shows that CAP is effective in reducing UTI recurrence in children with VUR.[58,59] Thus, CAP has

continued to be used in at least some patients with UTI and VUR, and recent survey found that most of the pediatric urologists recommend CAP for patients with high-grade VUR.[60]

Ongoing efforts have sought to determine potential consequences (positive and negative) of CAP, beyond its impact on UTI risk. Much has been made of the apparent lack of effect of CAP on incidence of new renal scarring in the RIVUR trial,[61] but it should be recalled that this trial was neither designed nor powered to look at renal scarring as an outcome. Circumstantial evidence suggests that CAP does indirectly reduce renal scarring risk through reduced incidence of UTI recurrence. For example, a secondary analysis of adherence data from the RIVUR trial found that those least adherent to prescribed CAP were 2.5 times more likely to have recurrent UTI versus the most adherent; furthermore, the least adherent patients were also at highest risk for renal scarring.[62] In addition, a different look at the RIVUR trial data confirmed that new renal scarring was more common among those with recurrent UTI and found that placebo was associated with a higher risk of recurrent UTI-associated new renal scarring (OR 3.1, 95% CI 1.0–8.8, $P = .04$) after adjusting for multiple additional factors.[63]

Concerns have been raised about potential impact of CAP on metabolic processes such as obesity and growth; however, Guidos and colleagues found that children with VUR who were on CAP did not have substantial changes in body mass index or height, when controlling for prior exposure to treatment-dose antibiotics and age.[64] Similarly, secondary analysis of RIVUR trial data showed no evidence that CAP affected weight gain or prevalence of obesity.[65] The impact of CAP on the microbiome has also been raised as a concern. The evidence here is quite limited, with some studies suggesting that CAP does not have a significant effect on gut microbial diversity,[66,67] whereas another suggested that changes in the microbiome do occur with CAP.[68] The clinical consequences of such changes are unknown.

The potential impact of CAP on antimicrobial resistance patterns has been a consistent concern in recent years. A study of RIVUR trial data showed that resistance to the agent used for CAP (trimethoprim-sulfamethoxazole) was significantly more common among those receiving CAP versus those on placebo, when UTI occurred (76% vs 28% of infections were resistant, among those with recurrent UTI); however, because CAP reduced the overall number of recurrent infections, there was no significant difference between groups in the overall proportion who experienced *resistant* recurrent UTI (9% of treatment group vs 6% of placebo group, OR = 1.46, 95% CI: 0.80–2.6).[69] Interestingly, resistance decreased over the course of the 2-year RIVUR study period, even in the CAP treatment group. Other studies have found mixed results. Selekman and colleagues compiled data from several randomized trials and found that among those with UTI, those with CAP were more likely to have a multidrug-resistant UTI (33% vs 6%, P < .001; OR 6.4, 95% CI: 2.7–15.6).[70]

One common clinical question is whether the resistance profile of the index infection should be used to determine choice of agent prescribed for CAP. A secondary study of RIVUR trial data showed that trimethoprim-sulfamethoxazole was equally effective regardless of whether the index infection was resistant or susceptible to trimethoprim-sulfamethoxazole.[69] However, a much smaller retrospective study found that breakthrough UTI was more common if the index UTI was resistant to trimethoprim-sulfamethoxazole when it was used for CAP.[71]

Alternatives to traditional antimicrobial agents for prevention of recurrent UTI are attractive in that they may avoid some of the undesirable aspects of these medications. Prophylaxis with probiotic agents was studied in a randomized trial in children with structurally normal urinary tract after first febrile UTI and found to be superior to placebo in preventing recurrence over 18 months.[72] Whether such agents are superior or equivalent to traditional antimicrobial prophylaxis remains to be studied.

Concerns about CAP use have also driven efforts to be more selective in use of this intervention. Analogous to efforts discussed earlier to identify subgroups of children with UTI who are most likely to have VUR on VCUG, efforts to develop models to identify children with VUR who are most likely to benefit from CAP have also been reported. The ultimate goal is to enable selective CAP use in those children who will have recurrent UTI without CAP, but no breakthrough UTI with CAP; those who will have recurrent UTI regardless of CAP use may be counseled to proceed with antireflux surgery as primary therapy, whereas those who will not have recurrent UTI regardless of CAP could be observed expectantly. Hidas and colleagues used logistic regression to predict 2-year probability of breakthrough UTI.[73] Risk factors included VUR grade, female gender, circumcision status, initial presentation after UTI, and bowel-bladder dysfunction (BBD), and the model showed the 2-year risk for breakthrough UTI was 8.6%, 26%, and 62.5% for low-, intermediate-, and high-risk groups, respectively.[73] Similarly, the group at Iowa published a series of

models demonstrating risk factors for breakthrough UTI, including dilating VUR, reflux occurring at low bladder volumes, BBD, and history of recurrent or febrile UTI associated with breakthrough UTI, with a model AUC of 0.755[74]; this same group further identified UDR as a predictive factor independent of reflux grade.[14,75] Comparing VUR Index, UDR, and reflux grade for prediction of breakthrough UTI, this group also found that both VUR Index and UDR were superior to reflux grade alone.[76]

As with VUR prediction, advanced analytics techniques have also been applied to the question of CAP utility, to identify those most likely to benefit. Bertsimas and colleagues used a machine learning model to analyze data from the RIVUR trial to predict such children, with factors including VUR grade, serum creatinine, race/gender, UTI symptoms (fever/dysuria), and weight percentiles; AUC of the prediction model was 0.82 (95% CI: 0.74–0.87).[77] Such advanced analytic techniques may help us to become more selective instead of using a one-size-fits-all approach to CAP.

TREATMENT OF VESICOURETERAL REFLUX: ANTIREFLUX SURGERY

Surgical intervention for VUR is indicated for patients who fail more conservative measures in order to reduce the incidence of febrile UTI and protect the upper urinary tract from damage. Open ureteral reimplantation (OUR) has historically been the gold standard in surgical management of VUR, with a high success rate and low complication rate. However, less invasive alternatives have long been sought; currently these include robotic-assisted laparoscopic ureteral reimplantation (RALUR) or endoscopic injection management as viable alternatives.

After its initial introduction as a surgical method in the early 2000s, RALUR has gained popularity, but in the United States remains an option limited to certain centers and patient subgroups. A 2016 review of the Kids' Inpatient Database showed that the proportion of ureteral reimplantation cases performed robotically increased from 0.3% in 2000 to 6.3% in 2012.[78] Although the availability and economics associated with robotic surgery (particularly in the pediatric setting) have played a role in limiting dissemination, perhaps the greatest hindrance has been concerns about efficacy and complications. There have been several studies, including multicenter studies, showing reduced VUR resolution and increased complications compared with OUR, whereas presumed advantages related to postoperative pain, hospital length of stay, and cosmesis were less clinically significant.[79] The retrospective multiinstitutional experience of Grimsby and colleagues found an overall clinical success of 72%, with 10% of patients having a complication and 11% needing to undergo reoperation.[80] Wang and colleagues reviewed the Nationwide Inpatient Sample database (1998–2012) and found that although RALUR had shorter length of stay (1.0 vs 1.8 days, $P < .001$), the approached was also associated with both higher costs and a higher incidence of postoperative urinary complications including UTIs, urinary retention, and renal injury (OR 3.1, $P = .02$).[81] Similarly, a review of the Premier Hospital Database at 17 hospitals in which both types of surgeries were performed between 2003 and 2013 found that incidence of any 90-day complication was significantly higher in the RALUR group (OR 3.17, $P = .0037$), and median hospital cost was higher, which is persistent after adjusting for demographic and regional factors.[82]

Not all evidence related to RALUR has been negative, however, and some studies have shown improvements in length of stay, pain control, recovery time, and surgical scar cosmesis. A 2014 single institution retrospective review of 50 patients that underwent RALUR showed 88% VUR resolution and 10% complication,[83] and a prospective multiinstitutional study from 2015 to 2017 of 143 patients showed an overall radiographic success of 93.8% and 94.1% for those with grade III to V VUR, with an overall ureteral complication incidence of 2.5%, which they argue is similar to reported outcomes for OUR and endoscopic injection.[84] A recent 2022 propensity score–matched analysis comparing OUR versus RALUR based on National Surgical Quality Improvement Program data found that RALUR patients tended to be older but reported 30-day complications showed no difference in readmission, reoperation, or extended hospital stay.[85] Some of the seemingly negative results with RALUR may be associated with the learning curve that tends to accompany any new procedure or technology; alternatively, the robotic approach may simply not be superior to OUR even in expert hands, due to the long-recognized low overall morbidity and high success of OUR. RALUR may be most beneficial for the older child or adolescent, where the morbidity of open abdominal surgery may be higher and the intrinsic advantages of minimally invasive reimplantation may be most evident.

Another alternative for the surgical management of VUR is endoscopic injection with a bulking agent. Initially described 4 decades ago, a variety of bulking agents have been reported over time, from tetrafluoroethylene to autologous cartilage.

Most recent clinical and research work has focused on a mixture of polysaccharide polymers, composed of dextranomer microspheres (a cross-linked polymer of dextran) and stabilized hyaluronic acid (DHA, marketed as Deflux). Initial work in the 1990s and early 2000s with DHA focused on demonstrating initial safety and efficacy, whereas in recent years there has been emphasis on optimizing the technique and refining specific indications for this treatment (as opposed to OUR). A 2010 systematic review by Routh and colleagues of 47 studies reported an overall success rate of 77% after 3 months; success depended on preoperative reflux grade, with lower grades of reflux being more successful, and varied widely between studies.[86]

In an effort to attempt to predict which patients would have DHA success, Payza and colleagues retrospectively reviewed 338 patients and found that higher ureteral diameter ratio (UDR, see earlier discussion) was associated with unsuccessful injection treatment and that UDR was more predictive of DHA failure than VUR grade alone.[87] Similarly, Baydilli and colleagues reviewed 200 patients who underwent DHA injection and found that failure was associated with early filling VUR on VCUG, UDR greater than 0.24, and delayed contrast drainage of the upper tract. Additional factors of presence of renal scarring, presence of bladder and bowel dysfunction, and history of febrile UTI were also associated with increased risk of DHA failure.[88] A 2017 review by Leung and colleagues of 53 children from 1995 to 2016 found that overall success rate was 57% after single injection after a median follow-up of 60 months and that lower VUR grade and absence of reflux were significant predictors of resolution on univariate analysis.[89]

The lower success of endoscopic injection in children with high-grade VUR was recognized early, and several groups have sought to delineate the true utility of DHA specifically for high-grade VUR. Friedmacher and colleagues reviewed their experience of DHA in high-grade VUR of 518 girls and 333 boys after a median follow-up of 8.5 years (range 6 months–16 years), and found an overall reflux resolution rate of 69.5% after first injection, with an additional 20.1% resolving after a second injection.[90] A 2020 retrospective review by Stenbäck and colleagues of their experience using DHA in grade IV patients found that 75% of those treated did not need to undergo ureteral reimplantation over their follow-up period and that injection success may have been attributable to injection technique.[91]

It has been argued by certain groups that VUR resolution is not the outcome that truly matters in most patients who undergo antireflux procedures; rather, it is absence of recurrent febrile UTI that is the true goal of treatment and that by this metric DHA injection is highly successful.[92] Adverse events related to endoscopic treatment with DHA have been recognized but seem to be relatively uncommon. Obstruction at the ureterovesical junction does occur in isolated instances, and some of these cases may be silent and progressive[93–95]; however, it seems that these events are infrequent. There have also been questions raised about the durability of DHA treatment, with reports of recurrence of VUR on long-term follow-up despite initial success, and there is debate about whether and for how long patients need to be followed after endoscopic treatment.[96] There have also been reports of calcification of DHA implants which can create the appearance of urolithiasis on imaging studies, particularly CT scans.[97] Despite these issues, however, DHA is a widely used and generally safe treatment, with acceptable success particularly for low-grade VUR; its utility as a treatment of high-grade VUR continues to be debated, particularly in light of the high standard established with OUR.

Although DHA is the most common bulking agent used at this time, other agents have been developed as alternatives, including polyacrylate-polyalcohol copolymer (PPC) and polyacrylamide hydrogel (PAHG). A review by Starmer and colleagues found that "current reports suggest PPC confers a higher resolution rate of VUR and PAHG confers comparable resolution rates" compared with DHA.[98] A randomized clinical trial comparing PPC with DHA injection outcomes at a median follow-up of 27.6 months found that PPC and DHA had similar outcomes but that subsequent OUR after failed injection treatment was more difficult in the PPC group.[99] As of early 2023, PPC and PAHG are not Food and Drug Administration approved in the United States for endoscopic treatment of VUR.

Urologists also continue to refine techniques of OUR to reduce its already low morbidity. Some centers have performed extravesical OUR on an outpatient basis and through smaller inguinal incisions.[100–102] Although not changing the basic surgical technique, such efforts seek to improve the patient and family experience and make an already well-tolerated procedure even less morbid.

SUMMARY

VUR is a complex condition ranging from a benign self-resolving radiographic finding to a severe disease associated with recurrent serious bacterial infection and chronic kidney disease. Investigation over the past 2 decades have improved our understanding of the natural history of VUR and helped identify those at higher risk of both VUR itself as well as its potential severe sequelae including recurrent pyelonephritis and acquired renal injury. Although CAP has been demonstrated to be effective in reducing the risk of recurrent UTI in children with VUR, efforts continue to identify those children most likely to benefit from CAP and to minimize adverse consequences such as resistant infection; the role of CAP in preventing renal scarring remains in question. New advanced analytic tools including artificial intelligence and machine learning have the potential to distill large volumes of granular data into practical tools that clinicians can use to guide diagnosis and management decisions for their patients and to identify specific patient most likely to benefit from diagnosis. Surgical treatment, when indicated, remains highly effective and is associated with low morbidity. Urologists nonetheless continue to refine techniques to become less invasive and better tolerated.

CLINICS CARE POINTS

- Despite increased understanding of the natural history of VUR, debate persists on key aspects of care, including when to perform diagnostic imaging and which patients benefit from continuous antibiotic prophylaxis.

- VCUG should be considered in children after initial febrile UTI if the ultrasound is abnormal, if the UTI was caused by a pathogen other than E coli, or if there is a family history of VUR and/or chronic kidney disease (CKD); all children should undergo VCUG after recurrent febrile UTI.

- Delayed treatment of febrile UTI, and recurrent febrile UTI, are associated with increased risk of renal scarring and CKD.

- Predictive models, including advanced analytic tools such as artificial intelligence and machine learning, have the potential to distill large volumes of granular data into practical tools that clinicians can use to guide diagnosis and management decisions for their patients with VUR.

DISCLOSURE

The authors have no commercial or financial conflicts of interest to disclose. E.M. Bortnick is a research fellow supported by an NIH, United

States T32 grant. This played no role in any aspect of manuscript design, manuscript preparation, or submission.

REFERENCES

1. Medical versus surgical treatment of primary vesicoureteral reflux: a prospective international reflux study in children. J Urol 1981;125(3):277–83.
2. Bailey R. Vesicoureteric reflux in healthy infants and children. In: Hodson J, Kincaid-Smith P, editors. Reflux Nephropathy. NY: Masson; 1979. p. 59–61.
3. Zorc JJ, Levine DA, Platt SL, et al. Clinical and demographic factors associated with urinary tract infection in young febrile infants. Pediatrics 2005; 116(3):644–8.
4. Chand DH, Rhoades T, Poe SA, et al. Incidence and severity of vesicoureteral reflux in children related to age, gender, race and diagnosis. J Urol 2003;170(4 Pt 2):1548–50.
5. Weiss R, Tamminen-Möbius T, Koskimies O, et al. Characteristics at entry of children with severe primary vesicoureteral reflux recruited for a multicenter, international therapeutic trial comparing medical and surgical management. The International Reflux Study in Children. J Urol 1992;148(5 Pt 2):1644–9.
6. RIVUR Trial Investigators, Hoberman A, Greenfield SP, et al. Antimicrobial prophylaxis for children with vesicoureteral reflux. N Engl J Med 2014;370(25):2367–76.
7. Capozza N, Gulia C, Heidari Bateni Z, et al. Vesicoureteral reflux in infants: what do we know about the gender prevalence by age? Eur Rev Med Pharmacol Sci 2017;21(23):5321–9.
8. Shaikh N, Lee MC, Stokes LR, et al. Reassessment of the Role of Race in Calculating the Risk for Urinary Tract Infection: A Systematic Review and Meta-analysis. JAMA Pediatr 2022;176(6):569–75.
9. Estrada CR, Passerotti CC, Graham DA, et al. Nomograms for predicting annual resolution rate of primary vesicoureteral reflux: results from 2,462 children. J Urol 2009;182(4):1535–41.
10. Kirsch AJ, Arlen AM, Leong T, et al. Vesicoureteral reflux index (VURx): a novel tool to predict primary reflux improvement and resolution in children less than 2 years of age. J Pediatr Urol 2014;10(6): 1249–54.
11. Arlen AM, Garcia-Roig M, Weiss AD, et al. Vesicoureteral Reflux Index: 2-Institution Analysis and Validation. J Urol 2016;195(4 Pt 2):1294–9.
12. Garcia-Roig M, Ridley DE, McCracken C, et al. Vesicoureteral Reflux Index: Predicting Primary Vesicoureteral Reflux Resolution in Children Diagnosed after Age 24 Months. J Urol 2017;197(4): 1150–7.
13. Cooper CS, Birusingh KK, Austin JC, et al. Distal ureteral diameter measurement objectively predicts vesicoureteral reflux outcome. J Pediatr Urol 2013;9(1):99–103.
14. Arlen AM, Kirsch AJ, Leong T, et al. Validation of the ureteral diameter ratio for predicting early spontaneous resolution of primary vesicoureteral reflux. J Pediatr Urol 2017;13(4):383.e1–6.
15. Nguyen HT, Herndon CDA, Cooper C, et al. The Society for Fetal Urology consensus statement on the evaluation and management of antenatal hydronephrosis. J Pediatr Urol 2010;6(3):212–31.
16. Nguyen HT, Benson CB, Bromley B, et al. Multidisciplinary consensus on the classification of prenatal and postnatal urinary tract dilation (UTD classification system). J Pediatr Urol 2014;10(6): 982–98.
17. Lee RS, Cendron M, Kinnamon DD, et al. Antenatal hydronephrosis as a predictor of postnatal outcome: a meta-analysis. Pediatrics 2006;118(2): 586–93.
18. Braga LH, Farrokhyar F, D'Cruz J, et al. Risk factors for febrile urinary tract infection in children with prenatal hydronephrosis: a prospective study. J Urol 2015;193(5 Suppl):1766–71.
19. Nelson CP, Lee RS, Trout AT, et al. The association of postnatal urinary tract dilation risk score with clinical outcomes. J Pediatr Urol 2019;15(4):341. e1–6.
20. Hwang HH, Cho MH, Ko CW. The necessity of voiding cystourethrography in children with prenatally diagnosed hydronephrosis. J Int Med Res 2011; 39(2):603–8.
21. Coelho GM, Bouzada MCF, Lemos GS, et al. Risk factors for urinary tract infection in children with prenatal renal pelvic dilatation. J Urol 2008; 179(1):284–9.
22. Zareba P, Lorenzo AJ, Braga LH. Risk factors for febrile urinary tract infection in infants with prenatal hydronephrosis: comprehensive single center analysis. J Urol 2014;191(5 Suppl):1614–8.
23. Kurtz MP, Nelson CP. Urology Mythbusters: should hydronephrosis grade be used to decide which newborns should undergo voiding cystourethrogram? J Pediatr Urol 2019;15(1):93–6.
24. Practice parameter: the diagnosis, treatment, and evaluation of the initial urinary tract infection in febrile infants and young children. American Academy of Pediatrics. Committee on Quality Improvement. Subcommittee on Urinary Tract Infection. Pediatrics 1999;103(4 Pt 1):843–52.
25. Subcommittee on Urinary Tract Infection, Steering Committee on Quality Improvement and Management, Roberts KB. Urinary tract infection: clinical practice guideline for the diagnosis and management of the initial UTI in febrile infants and children 2 to 24 months. Pediatrics 2011;128(3):595–610.

26. National Collaborating Centre for Women's and Children's Health (UK). Urinary tract infection in children: diagnosis, treatment and long-term management. RCOG Press; 2007. Available at: http://www.ncbi.nlm.nih.gov/books/NBK50606/. Accessed 3 February, 2023.

27. Wan J, Skoog SJ, Hulbert WC, et al. Section on Urology response to new Guidelines for the diagnosis and management of UTI. Pediatrics 2012; 129(4):e1051–3.

28. Nelson CP, Johnson EK, Logvinenko T, et al. Ultrasound as a screening test for genitourinary anomalies in children with UTI. Pediatrics 2014;133(3): e394–403.

29. Gaither TW, Selekman R, Kazi DS, et al. Cost-Effectiveness of Screening Ultrasound after a First, Febrile Urinary Tract Infection in Children Age 2-24 Months. J Pediatr 2020;216:73–81.e1.

30. Pennesi M, Amoroso S, Pennesi G, et al. Is ultrasonography mandatory in all children at their first febrile urinary tract infection? Pediatr Nephrol Berl Ger 2021;36(7):1809–16.

31. 't Hoen LA, Bogaert G, Radmayr C, et al. Update of the EAU/ESPU guidelines on urinary tract infections in children. J Pediatr Urol 2021;17(2): 200–7.

32. Arlen AM, Merriman LS, Kirsch JM, et al. Early effect of American Academy of Pediatrics Urinary Tract Infection Guidelines on radiographic imaging and diagnosis of vesicoureteral reflux in the emergency room setting. J Urol 2015;193(5 Suppl): 1760–5.

33. Lee T, Ellimoottil C, Marchetti KA, et al. Impact of Clinical Guidelines on Voiding Cystourethrogram Use and Vesicoureteral Reflux Incidence. J Urol 2018;199(3):831–6.

34. Ming JM, Lee LC, Chua ME, et al. Population-based trend analysis of voiding cystourethrogram ordering practices in a single-payer healthcare system before and after the release of evaluation guidelines. J Pediatr Urol 2019;15(2):152.e7.

35. Jacobson DL, Shannon R, Cheng EY, et al. Adherence to the 2011 American Academy of Pediatrics Urinary Tract Infection Guidelines for Voiding Cystourethrogram Ordering by Clinician Specialty. Urology 2019;126:180–6.

36. Lee T, Varda BK, Venna A, et al. Changes in Clinical Presentation and Renal Outcomes among Children with Febrile Urinary Tract Infection: 2005 vs 2015. J Urol 2021;205(6):1764–9.

37. Mathias S, Greenbaum LA, Shubha AM, et al. Risk factors for renal scarring and clinical morbidity in children with high-grade and low-grade primary vesicoureteral reflux. J Pediatr Urol 2022;18(2): 225.e1–8.

38. Yılmaz İ, Peru H, Yılmaz FH, et al. Association of vesicoureteral reflux and renal scarring in urinary tract infections. Arch Argent Pediatr 2018;116(4): e542–7.

39. Shaikh N, Haralam MA, Kurs-Lasky M, et al. Association of Renal Scarring With Number of Febrile Urinary Tract Infections in Children. JAMA Pediatr 2019;173(10):949–52.

40. Doğan ÇS, Koyun NS, Aksoy GK, et al. Delayed diagnosis of primary vesicoureteral reflux in children with recurrent urinary tract infections: Diagnostic approach and renal outcomes. Turk J Urol 2018;44(6):498–502.

41. Ergun R, Sekerci CA, Tanidir Y, et al. Abnormal DMSA renal scan findings and associated factors in older children with vesicoureteral reflux. Int Urol Nephrol 2021;53(10):1963–8.

42. Shaikh N, Mattoo TK, Keren R, et al. Early Antibiotic Treatment for Pediatric Febrile Urinary Tract Infection and Renal Scarring. JAMA Pediatr 2016; 170(9):848–54.

43. Alberici I, La Manna A, Pennesi M, et al. First urinary tract infections in children: the role of the risk factors proposed by the Italian recommendations. Acta Paediatr Oslo Nor 2019;108(3):544–50.

44. Kobayashi Y, Mishina H, Michihata N, et al. Indication for voiding cystourethrography during first urinary tract infection. Pediatr Int Off J Jpn Pediatr Soc 2019;61(6):595–600.

45. Roesch J, Harms M, Berger C, et al. Targeted Indication of Imaging for Detection of Vesicoureteric Reflux after Pediatric Febrile Urinary Tract Infections Based on a Multiparametric Computational Tool. Indian J Pediatr 2020;87(12):1001–8.

46. Breinbjerg A, Jørgensen CS, Frøkiær J, et al. Risk factors for kidney scarring and vesicoureteral reflux in 421 children after their first acute pyelonephritis, and appraisal of international guidelines. Pediatr Nephrol Berl Ger 2021;36(9):2777–87. https://doi.org/10.1007/s00467-021-05042-7.

47. Klubdaeng A, Chaiyapak T, Sumboonnanonda A, et al. Model for predicting high-grade vesicoureteral reflux in young children presenting with febrile urinary tract infection. J Pediatr Urol 2022;18(4): 518–24. https://doi.org/10.1016/j.jpurol.2022.06.006.

48. Advanced Analytics Group of Pediatric Urology and ORC Personalized Medicine Group. Targeted Workup after Initial Febrile Urinary Tract Infection: Using a Novel Machine Learning Model to Identify Children Most Likely to Benefit from Voiding Cystourethrogram. J Urol 2019;202(1):144–52. https://doi.org/10.1097/JU.0000000000000186.

49. Aggarwal VK, Verrier Jones K. Vesicoureteric reflux: screening of first degree relatives. Arch Dis Child 1989;64(11):1538–41. https://doi.org/10.1136/adc.64.11.1538.

50. Skoog SJ, Peters CA, Arant BS, et al. Pediatric Vesicoureteral Reflux Guidelines Panel Summary

Report: Clinical Practice Guidelines for Screening Siblings of Children With Vesicoureteral Reflux and Neonates/Infants With Prenatal Hydronephrosis. J Urol 2010;184(3):1145–51.

51. Routh JC, Grant FD, Kokorowski P, et al. Costs and consequences of universal sibling screening for vesicoureteral reflux: decision analysis. Pediatrics 2010;126(5):865–71.

52. Nelson CP, Finkelstein JA, Logvinenko T, et al. Incidence of Urinary Tract Infection Among Siblings of Children With Vesicoureteral Reflux. Acad Pediatr 2016;16(5):489–95.

53. Darge K. Voiding urosonography with ultrasound contrast agents for the diagnosis of vesicoureteric reflux in children. I. Procedure. Pediatr Radiol 2008;38(1):40–53.

54. Darge K. Voiding urosonography with US contrast agents for the diagnosis of vesicoureteric reflux in children. II. Comparison with radiological examinations. Pediatr Radiol 2008;38(1):54–63. quiz 126-127.

55. Paltiel HJ, Barnewolt CE, Chow JS, et al. Accuracy of contrast-enhanced voiding urosonography using Optison™ for diagnosis of vesicoureteral reflux in children. J Pediatr Urol 2023;19(1):135.e1–8.

56. Sofia C, Solazzo A, Cattafi A, et al. Contrast-enhanced voiding urosonography in the assessment of vesical-ureteral reflux: the time has come. Radiol Med 2021;126(7):901–9.

57. Smellie JM, Grüneberg RN, Leakey A, et al. Long-term low-dose co-trimoxazole in prophylaxis of childhood urinary tract infection: clinical aspects. Br Med J 1976;2(6029):203–6.

58. Wang HHS, Gbadegesin RA, Foreman JW, et al. Efficacy of antibiotic prophylaxis in children with vesicoureteral reflux: systematic review and meta-analysis. J Urol 2015;193(3):963–9.

59. Williams G, Craig JC. Long-term antibiotics for preventing recurrent urinary tract infection in children. Cochrane Database Syst Rev 2019;4(4): CD001534.

60. Hamdy RF, Pohl HG, Forster CS. Antibiotic Prophylaxis Prescribing Patterns of Pediatric Urologists for Children with Vesicoureteral Reflux and other Congenital Anomalies of the Kidney and Urinary Tract. Urology 2020;136:225–30.

61. Roberts KB. AAP Subcommittee on Urinary Tract Infection. Antimicrobial prophylaxis for children with vesicoureteral reflux. N Engl J Med 2014; 371(11):1071.

62. Gaither TW, Copp HL. Antimicrobial prophylaxis for urinary tract infections: implications for adherence assessment. J Pediatr Urol 2019;15(4):387.e1–8.

63. Wang HH, Kurtz M, Logvinenko T, et al. Why Does Prevention of Recurrent Urinary Tract Infection not Result in Less Renal Scarring? A Deeper Dive into the RIVUR Trial. J Urol 2019;202(2):400–5.

64. Guidos PJ, Arlen AM, Leong T, et al. Impact of continuous low-dose antibiotic prophylaxis on growth in children with vesicoureteral reflux. J Pediatr Urol 2018;14(4):325.e1–7.

65. Edmonson MB, Eickhoff JC. Weight Gain and Obesity in Infants and Young Children Exposed to Prolonged Antibiotic Prophylaxis. JAMA Pediatr 2017;171(2):150–6.

66. Akagawa Y, Kimata T, Akagawa S, et al. Impact of Long-Term Low Dose Antibiotic Prophylaxis on Gut Microbiota in Children. J Urol 2020;204(6):1320–5.

67. Strasser C, Spindelboeck W, Kashofer K, et al. Low-dose antibiotic prophylaxis has no significant impact on the stability of the intestinal microbiome in children with urogenital tract malformations under 1 year of age. J Pediatr Urol 2020;16(4):456. e1–7.

68. Morello W, D'Amico F, Serafinelli J, et al. Low-Dose Antibiotic Prophylaxis Induces Rapid Modifications of the Gut Microbiota in Infants With Vesicoureteral Reflux. Front Pediatr 2021;9:674716.

69. Nelson CP, Hoberman A, Shaikh N, et al. Antimicrobial Resistance and Urinary Tract Infection Recurrence. Pediatrics 2016;137(4):e20152490.

70. Selekman RE, Shapiro DJ, Boscardin J, et al. Uropathogen Resistance and Antibiotic Prophylaxis: A Meta-analysis. Pediatrics 2018;142(1):e20180119.

71. Lee JN, Byeon KH, Woo MJ, et al. Susceptibility of the Index Urinary Tract Infection to Prophylactic Antibiotics Is a Predictive Factor of Breakthrough Urinary Tract Infection in Children with Primary Vesicoureteral Reflux Receiving Continuous Antibiotic Prophylaxis. J Korean Med Sci 2019;34(21):e156.

72. Sadeghi-Bojd S, Naghshizadian R, Mazaheri M, et al. Efficacy of Probiotic Prophylaxis After The First Febrile Urinary Tract Infection in Children With Normal Urinary Tracts. J Pediatr Infect Dis Soc 2020;9(3):305–10.

73. Hidas G, Billimek J, Nam A, et al. Predicting the Risk of Breakthrough Urinary Tract Infections: Primary Vesicoureteral Reflux. J Urol 2015;194(5): 1396–401.

74. Arlen AM, Alexander SE, Wald M, et al. Computer model predicting breakthrough febrile urinary tract infection in children with primary vesicoureteral reflux. J Pediatr Urol 2016;12(5):288.e1–5.

75. Troesch VL, Wald M, Bonnett MA, et al. The additive impact of the distal ureteral diameter ratio in predicting early breakthrough urinary tract infections in children with vesicoureteral reflux. J Pediatr Urol 2021;17(2):208.e1–5.

76. Arlen AM, Leong T, Wu CQ, et al. Predicting Breakthrough Urinary Tract Infection: Comparative Analysis of Vesicoureteral Reflux Index, Reflux Grade and Ureteral Diameter Ratio. J Urol 2020;204(3): 572–7.

77. Bertsimas D, Li M, Estrada C, et al. Selecting Children with Vesicoureteral Reflux Who are Most Likely to Benefit from Antibiotic Prophylaxis: Application of Machine Learning to RIVUR. J Urol 2021; 205(4):1170–9.

78. Bowen DK, Faasse MA, Liu DB, et al. Use of Pediatric Open, Laparoscopic and Robot-Assisted Laparoscopic Ureteral Reimplantation in the United States: 2000 to 2012. J Urol 2016;196(1):207–12.

79. Cannon GM, Ost MC. Robot-Assisted Laparoscopic Extravesical Ureteral Reimplantation for Primary Vesicoureteral Reflux in Children. J Urol 2017; 197(6):1379–81.

80. Grimsby GM, Dwyer ME, Jacobs MA, et al. Multiinstitutional review of outcomes of robot-assisted laparoscopic extravesical ureteral reimplantation. J Urol 2015;193(5 Suppl):1791–5.

81. Wang HHS, Tejwani R, Cannon GM, et al. Open versus minimally invasive ureteroneocystostomy: A population-level analysis. J Pediatr Urol 2016; 12(4):232.e1–6.

82. Kurtz MP, Leow JJ, Varda BK, et al. Robotic versus open pediatric ureteral reimplantation: Costs and complications from a nationwide sample. J Pediatr Urol 2016;12(6):408.e1–6.

83. Akhavan A, Avery D, Lendvay TS. Robot-assisted extravesical ureteral reimplantation: outcomes and conclusions from 78 ureters. J Pediatr Urol 2014;10(5):864–8.

84. Boysen WR, Akhavan A, Ko J, et al. Prospective multicenter study on robot-assisted laparoscopic extravesical ureteral reimplantation (RALUR-EV): Outcomes and complications. J Pediatr Urol 2018;14(3):262.e1–6.

85. Chalfant V, Riveros C, Stec AA. Open versus minimally invasive ureteroneocystostomy: trends and outcomes in a NSQIP-P cohort. J Robot Surg 2022. https://doi.org/10.1007/s11701-022-01437-2.

86. Routh JC, Inman BA, Reinberg Y. Dextranomer/hyaluronic acid for pediatric vesicoureteral reflux: systematic review. Pediatrics 2010;125(5):1010–9.

87. Payza AD, Hoşgör M, Serdaroğlu E, et al. Can distal ureteral diameter measurement predict primary vesicoureteral reflux clinical outcome and success of endoscopic injection? J Pediatr Urol 2019;15(5):515.e1–8.

88. Baydilli N, Selvi I, Pinarbasi AS, et al. Additional VCUG-related parameters for predicting the success of endoscopic injection in children with primary vesicoureteral reflux. J Pediatr Urol 2021; 17(1):68.e1–8.

89. Leung L, Chan IHY, Chung PHY, et al. Endoscopic injection for primary vesicoureteric reflux: Predictors of resolution and long term efficacy. J Pediatr Surg 2017;52(12):2066–9.

90. Friedmacher F, Colhoun E, Puri P. Endoscopic Injection of Dextranomer/Hyaluronic Acid as First Line Treatment in 851 Consecutive Children with High Grade Vesicoureteral Reflux: Efficacy and Long-Term Results. J Urol 2018;200(3):650–5.

91. Stenbäck A, Olafsdottir T, Sköldenberg E, et al. Proprietary non-animal stabilized hyaluronic acid/dextranomer gel (NASHA/Dx) for endoscopic treatment of grade IV vesicoureteral reflux: Long-term observational study. J Pediatr Urol 2020;16(3): 328.e1–9.

92. Kaye JD, Srinivasan AK, Delaney C, et al. Clinical and radiographic results of endoscopic injection for vesicoureteral reflux: defining measures of success. J Pediatr Urol 2012;8(3):297–303.

93. Chung JM, Park CS, Lee SD. Postoperative ureteral obstruction after endoscopic treatment for vesicoureteral reflux. Korean J Urol 2015;56(7):533–9.

94. Friedmacher F, Puri P. Ureteral Obstruction After Endoscopic Treatment of Vesicoureteral Reflux: Does the Type of Injected Bulking Agent Matter? Curr Urol Rep 2019;20(9):49.

95. García-Aparicio L, Rodo J, Palazon P, et al. Acute and delayed vesicoureteral obstruction after endoscopic treatment of primary vesicoureteral reflux with dextranomer/hyaluronic acid copolymer: why and how to manage. J Pediatr Urol 2013;9(4): 493–7.

96. Fuentes S, Gómez-Fraile A, Carrillo-Arroyo I, et al. Factors involved in the late failure of endoscopic treatment of vesicoureteral reflux. Actas Urol Esp 2018;42(5):331–7.

97. Cerwinka WH, Kaye JD, Scherz HC, et al. Radiologic features of implants after endoscopic treatment of vesicoureteral reflux in children. AJR Am J Roentgenol 2010;195(1):234–40.

98. Starmer B, McAndrew F, Corbett H. A review of novel STING bulking agents. J Pediatr Urol 2019; 15(5):484–90.

99. García-Aparicio L, Blázquez-Gómez E, Martin O, et al. Randomized clinical trial between polyacrylate-polyalcohol copolymer (PPC) and dextranomer-hyaluronic acid copolymer (Dx/HA) as bulking agents for endoscopic treatment of primary vesicoureteral reflux (VUR). World J Urol 2018;36(10):1651–6.

100. Putman S, Wicher C, Wayment R, et al. Unilateral extravesical ureteral reimplantation in children performed on an outpatient basis. J Urol 2005;174(5): 1987–9. discussion 1989-1990.

101. Yap M, Nseyo U, Din H, et al. Unilateral extravesical ureteral reimplantation via inguinal incision for the correction of vesicoureteral reflux: a 10-year experience. Int Braz J Urol Off J Braz Soc Urol 2017; 43(5):917–24.

102. Wiygul J, Palmer LS. The inguinal approach to extravesical ureteral reimplantation is safe, effective, and efficient. J Pediatr Urol 2011;7(3):257–60.

Exstrophy-Epispadias Complex

Ted Lee, MD, MSc[a,b,*], Joseph Borer, MD[a,b]

KEYWORDS

- Epispadias • Bladder exstrophy • Cloacal exstrophy • OEIS

KEY POINTS

- Each entity within the EEC spectrum presents with a unique set of pathologic conditions that must be approached with care and caution.
- Timely diagnosis and appropriate counseling during the perinatal period are imperative.
- Reconstruction should be performed by an experienced surgeon and team familiar with the intricacies of EEC anatomy and sequelae of major reconstruction.
- Regardless of initial surgical approach, patients affected by EEC frequently struggle with long-term incontinence and sexual dysfunction that need to be addressed through an individualized approach, taking into consideration both psychosocial and anatomic factors.

INTRODUCTION

Exstrophy-epispadias complex (EEC) encompasses a spectrum of disorders with lower abdominal midline malformations, including epispadias, bladder exstrophy, and cloacal exstrophy, also known as Omphalocele–Exstrophy–Imperforate Anus–Spinal Anomalies Complex (OEIS). In this review, the authors discuss the epidemiology, embryologic cause, prenatal findings, phenotypic characteristics, and management strategies of these 3 conditions. The primary focus is to summarize outcomes pertaining to each condition.

DISCUSSION
Epidemiology

The incidence of EEC differs by subtype. The incidence of epispadias is estimated to be 2.4 per 100,000 with a male-to-female ratio of 1.4:1.[1,2] Notably, historic studies may have overestimated male-to-female ratios owing to missed or delayed diagnosis of epispadias in incontinent female patients.[3] The incidence of bladder exstrophy is approximately 4.0 per 100,000 with a male-to-female ratio of around 2.4:1.[1,4–7] The prevalence of OEIS is estimated to be 0.5 to 1 per 100,000,

but the true incidence may be higher due to frequency of undiagnosed OEIS in stillbirths.[5,7–10] OEIS appears to occur more frequently in girls than in boys.[2,5,10]

Embryologic Cause

Several theories have been proposed to explain the embryologic origins of EEC. One theory is cloacal membrane overdevelopment that prevents medial migration of the mesoderm. This results in eventual rupture of the cloacal membrane owing to absent mesenchymal support. If the rupture of the cloacal membrane occurs early in gestation before the presence of the urorectal septum, this results in a lateral enterovesical fistula seen in OEIS. Conversely, if the rupture of the cloacal membrane occurs later in development after medial migration of the mesenchyme in the anterior abdominal wall but not the urethra, it will result in epispadias.[11–14] Another theory involves abnormalities in temporal-spatial development of the pelvic bone and bladder. Maldevelopment of the bony pelvis prevents midline approximation of pelvic organs, resulting in EEC.[15,16] Other hypotheses involve fusion of midline below the cloacal membrane and abnormal caudal insertion

a Department of Urology, Boston Children's Hospital, 300 Longwood Avenue Boston, MA 02115, USA;
b Department of Surgery (Urology), Harvard Medical School, Boston, MA, USA
* Corresponding author.
E-mail address: Ted.Lee@childrens.harvard.edu

Urol Clin N Am 50 (2023) 403–414
https://doi.org/10.1016/j.ucl.2023.04.004
0094-0143/23/© 2023 Elsevier Inc. All rights reserved.

of the body stalk that prevents midline mesenchymal approximation.[17–19]

Prenatal Findings

Bladder exstrophy and OEIS can be diagnosed with ultrasonography or MRI during the fetal period.[20–22] Four common prenatal ultrasound findings for fetuses with bladder exstrophy are an unvisualized bladder, lower abdominal mass, low umbilical insertion, and abnormal widening of the iliac crests.[22] In male fetuses, a small phallus with anteriorly displaced scrotum can be seen.[22] Fetuses affected by OEIS often have concomitant findings involving the gastrointestinal tract and spine. Bladder exstrophy and OEIS can further be differentiated by the location of the umbilical cord insertion relative to the abdominal wall defect. An inferior insertion is suggestive of OEIS.[21] Recent review of a multi-institutional EEC database revealed a prenatal diagnosis rate of 47% in bladder exstrophy and 82% in OEIS over the past 20 years.[23]

Phenotypic Characteristics

Epispadias
In epispadias, the inner lining of the urethra lays flat and exposed on the dorsal surface (**Fig. 1**). Subtypes of epispadias are defined by the physical location of the urethral meatus. In male patients, epispadias is classified as glanular epispadias if the meatal location is glanular, penile epispadias if the opening is within the penile shaft, and penopubic epispadias if the defect is more proximally located within the penopubic junction. In female patients, epispadias is categorized as vesicular if the urethra is mainly normal but altered in relation to the clitoris, which is located inferior to the urethral opening. Subsymphyseal epispadias includes a defect in the anterior wall of the entire urethra for approximately one-half its length. Retropubic epispadias is the most severe form, in which the anterior wall defect spans the entirety of the urethra. It is common to refer distal meatal location as "mild" and more proximal meatal location as "severe" forms of epispadias. However, continence status and degree of bladder neck coaptation do not always correlate with the "severity" of epispadias.[7]

Bladder exstrophy
Typical findings include an open bladder plate in which the inner mucosal surface is exposed (**Figs. 2** and **3**). Bladder exstrophy is accompanied by epispadias. Additional anomalies include a low-set umbilicus, anteriorly displaced pelvic floor musculature, anteriorly displaced anus, externally rotated anterior and posterior pelvis, acetabular retroversion, and diastasis of the pubic symphysis. In male patients, separation of pubic bones and rotational deformities of the pelvic skeletal structures contribute to the short, pendular penis often accompanied by dorsal curvature.[24] In female patients, the vaginal orifice is typically anteriorly displaced and includes a more horizontal axis.[25]

Omphalocele–exstrophy–imperforate anus–spinal anomalies complex
OEIS is characterized by exstrophy of the urinary bladder and cecal plate through an abdominal wall defect, anal atresia, hypoplasia of the colon, omphalocele, and anomalous genitalia (**Fig. 4**). There may also be hypoplasia of the small intestine that could result in short gut syndrome. Pelvic bone abnormalities are typically more pronounced in OEIS relative to bladder exstrophy. The vertebral column (backbone) and spinal cord are abnormal in nearly all individuals, resulting in neurologic and lower-extremity impairments. There may also be associated abnormalities of one or both kidneys, such as impaired development, abnormal function or position, or absence of a kidney.[8,12]

Initial Surgical Management

Epispadias
Urgent intervention during the newborn period is not needed. Before surgery, assessment of dry intervals is essential during physical examination (eg, urinary leakage during Valsalva) and clinical history. Furthermore, appearance and functionality of the bladder neck are essential through the use of voiding cystourethrography, urodynamic studies, and cystoscopy. Depending on continence status and appearance of the bladder neck, surgical management ranges from isolated penile repair to concomitant bladder neck reconstruction, with or without pelvic bone osteotomies. There are 2 types of penile repairs that are commonly used. The first is the modified Cantwell-Ransley procedure, which includes partial disassembly of the penis, ventral transposition of the urethra, dorsal rotation and approximation of the corpora, and a reverse meatal advancement and glanuloplasty, also referred to as IPGAM.[26] The second is the Mitchell technique, which involves complete penile disassembly. Complete disassembly allows for tubularization of the entire length of the urethra.[27] The benefit of the Mitchell technique is improved ability to correct for dorsal chordee and increased penile length. However, this comes at the risk of compromised blood supply with more aggressive dissection and potential

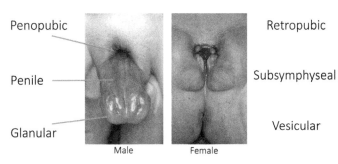

Penopubic

Penile

Glanular

Male   Female

Retropubic

Subsymphyseal

Vesicular

Fig. 1. Phenotypic characteristics of epispadias subtypes for male and female patients.

hypospadiac meatus.[28] Epispadias repairs are typically performed after 1 year of age to minimize risk of anesthesia but before toilet training age. Urethrocutaneous fistula is the most common complication, which occurs in 13% to 18% of cases.[29,30]

Bladder exstrophy

Following delivery, the initial plastic umbilical cord clamp should be exchanged for soft cloth umbilical tape or silk ligature to limit trauma to the exposed surface of the bladder. The bladder is covered with a nonadherent film of plastic wrap or a transparent adhesive dressing until bladder closure. There are many surgical techniques described, but there are three that are most commonly used today: Modern Staged Repair of Bladder Exstrophy (MSRE), Complete Primary Repair of Bladder Exstrophy (CPRE), and the Kelly repair, also referred to as radical soft tissue mobilization.[31–35]

MSRE was first introduced by Dr Bob Jeffs in the 1970s. The first stage involves abdominal wall, bladder, and posterior urethra closure typically during the first 72 hours of life. Osteotomy is performed if the closure occurs after the first 72 hours or if the pubic diastasis is greater than 4 cm. The second stage of MSRE includes epispadias repair at 6 months to 1 year of age. If bladder capacity is adequate and patient/family are ready for toilet training, the third stage of

bladder neck reconstruction and bilateral ureteral reimplantation is typically performed.[31,32] CPRE was first introduced by Dr Michael Mitchell in 1989. CPRE involves closure of the bladder, bladder neck, and urethra as a single unit at 6 to 8 weeks of age. The key motivation behind this technique is the earlier introduction of bladder outlet resistance, thus creating an environment that facilitates earlier bladder growth and development.[33] In the Kelly repair, the bladder is closed during the newborn period without attempts to bring the pubic bones into apposition. During the second step, a radical soft tissue mobilization is performed, completely mobilizing the corpora off the pubic bones and deeply incising through the pelvic floor laterally. The urethral plate is mobilized from the corporal bodies and moved below to iatrogenically create a penoscrotal hypospadias.[34] The theoretical benefit of the Kelly repair is the added penile length owing to proximal dissection of the corpora. However, this comes at the risk of damage to the neurovascular bundle and theoretical increased risk of damaging the blood supply to the penis. Complications involving any surgical approach include bladder dehiscence, penile ischemia, urethrocutaneous/vesicocutaneous fistula, bladder outlet stricture/obstruction, and urinary tract infections.[28]

Importantly, there has been a recent trend in delaying initial closure for bladder exstrophy. In a

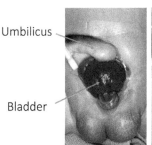
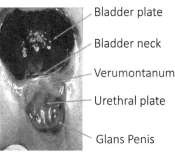

Umbilicus

Bladder

Bladder plate

Bladder neck

Verumontanum

Urethral plate

Glans Penis

Fig. 2. Phenotypic characteristics of bladder exstrophy in male patients.

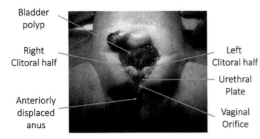

Fig. 3. Phenotypic characteristics of bladder exstrophy in female patients.

publicly available administrative database from 1999 to 2010, 75% of patients underwent primary closure within the first 3 days of life.[35] Since the 2010s, however, there has been a trend in delaying initial closure for bladder exstrophy beyond 4 weeks for both MSRE and CPRE.[36–38] Delays in initial closure appear to be safe.[39] The reasons for delayed closure include increased maternal bonding during the newborn period, accommodation of family schedules, and availability of orthopedic surgeons at the time of closure.[40] Given the importance of a successful initial surgical closure in long-term outcomes, complexity of the surgery, rarity of the condition, and safety of delayed closure, there has been a push within the bladder exstrophy community to concentrate bladder exstrophy–related care to designated "centers of excellence."[41] The same logic applies to management of epispadias and OEIS.

Omphalocele-exstrophy-imperforate anus-spinal anomalies complex

The initial goal of genitourinary reconstruction is to bring the 2 hemibladder plates together by excising the omphalocele and separating the cecal plate from bladder halves. The 2 bladder halves are approximated in the midline, and an end colostomy with or without a protective ileostomy is created. The second stage of the procedure is similar to reconstruction of bladder exstrophy, with steps including iliac osteotomies, bladder

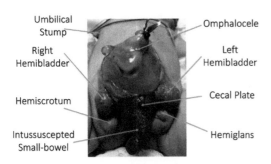

Fig. 4. Phenotypic characteristics of OEIS.

closure, urethroplasty, and reconstruction of external genitalia.[24] The second-stage procedure is typically performed before 1 year of age, but timing is largely dependent on the overall condition of the cloacal exstrophy patient, specifically, nutrition status and growth curve. In addition to the aforementioned complications involving bladder exstrophy closure, patients with OEIS undergoing second-stage repair are particularly at risk of increased abdominal/pelvic pressures following lower abdominal wall closure. This may result in decreased lung volumes, reduced chest wall compliance, compromised renal function, glans ischemia, and prolonged ileus.[42,43]

Continence Outcomes

There are significant challenges in reporting and interpreting continence outcomes in EEC owing to lack of standard definitions. The most commonly used definition is maintenance of dry periods of 3 or more hours during the day without stress incontinence, although others have used 2 or more hours.[44,45] As dry periods can vary heavily depending on positioning and degree of fluid consumption, others have used the concept of "mild" continence, defined as using 1 pad per day and persistent nocturnal enuresis.[46] For the purposes of this review, continence was defined as dry periods of 3 or more hours during the day unless specified otherwise.

Epispadias

The initial meatal location is loosely associated with the severity of incontinence. In other words, although there is higher likelihood of continence for individuals with more distal meatal location, there is still a significant portion of patients with distal meatal location that struggle with life-long incontinence. Review of the literature suggests that most patients with penopubic epispadias will require one or more bladder neck level procedures to achieve continence. Select patients with glanular or penile epispadias may need additional continence procedures, although it can be challenging to precisely predict which patients are at highest risk.

Several studies have reported continence outcomes in male epispadias. Kramer and Kelalis[47] reported 21 of 82 (26%) patients having complete continence preoperatively (12 of 12 glanular, 6 of 21 penile, and 3 of 49 penopubic). Thirty-two boys required bladder neck reconstruction, after which 22 of 32 (69%) patients developed continence. Mollard and colleagues[48] reported 14 patients with penopubic epispadias who underwent bladder neck reconstruction before any penile reconstruction, and 84% achieved continence after one or more continence procedures. More recently, Braga and colleagues[49] reported continence outcomes for 19 patients with incontinent penopubic epispadias. Thirteen of those patients who underwent Cantwell-Ransley epispadias repair alone remained incontinent. Four of 6 (67%) who underwent a more proximal dissection achieved dryness. Eleven of the 19 (58%) underwent one or more bladder neck procedures to achieve dryness, and 3 of 19 (16%) underwent augmentation cystoplasty. In another series of 26 boys (4 glanular, 8 penile, and 14 penopubic), glanular, penile, and penopubic epispadias had a 75%, 63%, and 64% rate of dry intervals greater than 2 hours, respectively.[7] Another series of 30 boys (3 glanular, 3 penile, 24 penopubic) demonstrated that 26 of 30 (86%) patients, including 2 with penile epispadias and 1 with glanular epispadias, required additional surgery for continence following initial epispadias repair, including bulking injections, bladder neck reconstruction, slings, or the Kelly procedure.[50]

Outcome studies for female epispadias patients is less common and smaller in sample size. Purves and colleagues[51] reported that 74% of those who underwent staged repair achieved daytime and nighttime continence. Mean times to daytime and nocturnal enuresis were 12 and 18 months, respectively. Cheikhelard and colleagues reported continence outcomes of 85% following a 1-stage repair, including bladder neck and pelvic floor reconstruction.[52] Suson and colleagues[53] reported 8 of 19 (42%) achieved continence following initial reconstructing, including perineal urethroplasty and feminizing genitoplasty early in infancy or when condition is identified. An additional 6 (32%) required bladder neck reconstruction to achieve continence, 2 of whom are requiring clean intermittent catheterization. Five (26%) required augmentation cystoplasty.

Bladder exstrophy

In addition to the lack of standard definitions and objective measures to accurately assess continence, there are several confounding factors that make it challenging to interpret continence outcomes in bladder exstrophy. There is significant variation in type and quality of bladder closure surgeries performed. Furthermore, many of the studies reporting continence outcomes fail to disclose in detail the number and type of procedures required to establish continence. Studies frequently do not distinguish patients within the EEC spectrum, fail to account for patients lost to follow-up, and include those too young to reasonably achieve continence within the denominator. Hence, only select studies were included in this review.

The largest and most recent case series for MSRE reports continence outcomes for 350 eligible patients (eg, continence data available at least 3 months following last continence procedure). Eighty of 350 (23%) were able to achieve continence while spontaneous voiding with bladder neck reconstruction alone. Overall, 432 patients in total underwent successful bladder closure and a urinary continence procedure with a median follow-up of 7.2 years. One hundred sixty-two of 432 (37%) underwent bladder neck reconstruction; 76 of 432 (18%) underwent bladder neck reconstruction with augmentation cystoplasty/continent catheterizable channel, and 173 of 432 (40%) underwent bladder neck closure with continent catheterizable channel. Following isolated bladder neck reconstruction, 64% achieved continence through either spontaneous voiding or clean intermittent catheterization. Interestingly, 61% of those who underwent bladder neck reconstruction with augmentation cystoplasty/continent catheterizable achieved continence. Greater than 90% of those who underwent bladder neck closure were continent.[54]

There are few studies reporting long-term continence outcomes following CPRE or Kelly technique owing to their relative recent introduction and uptake. Ellison and colleagues[55] reported continence outcomes in 29 patients following CPRE with mean follow-up of nearly 4 years. Overall, 5 of 29 (17%) patients achieved continence with initial surgery alone. Seven additional patients achieved continence with additional bladder neck reconstruction or bladder neck injection. Jarzebowski and colleagues[56] reported continence outcomes in 31 patients older than 4 years of age following repair with Kelly technique. Three of the 31 (10%) patients were voiding spontaneously with complete continence, and an additional 9 patients achieved partial continence with spontaneous voids.14

What is clear from these studies is that, regardless of technique, the rate of complete continence through voluntary voiding is quite low (10%–25%) following initial surgery alone. Additional surgeries, including bladder neck reconstruction, bladder neck closure, augmentation cystoplasty, and/or continent catheterizable channels, are required to improve continence. The low proportion of patients achieving continence through voluntary voiding may be due to relatively short follow-up times of the studies reporting continence outcomes, because some patients may gain continence over time through improved pelvic floor musculature, behavioral modifications, and prostatic growth in male patients. However, in a multi-institutional study that included 216 patients, nearly 90% underwent a bladder neck procedure with synchronous augmentation rate near 30% by age 18. The probability of bladder augmentation or urinary diversion was 15% by 5 years, 51% by 10 years, and 70% by 18 years, although the probability of augmentation or urinary diversion varied significantly between the 5 centers.[57]

Management of persistent continence should be highly individualized depending on each patient's anatomy and psychosocial situation. From an anatomic standpoint, the degree of bladder neck resistance and detrusor compliance/capacity should be carefully studied with cystoscopy, urodynamics, and imaging. Insufficient narrowing of the bladder neck will not result in necessary bladder outlet resistance to achieve continence. On the contrary, significant bladder outlet resistance in the setting of low-compliant/small-capacity bladder will lead to high-pressure voiding, resulting in urinary tract infection, epididymitis, incomplete emptying, stone formation, and upper tract damage.[58]

If the bladder neck appears narrow and bladder capacity/compliance is adequate in a preteen child with persistent incontinence, it may be prudent to wait for puberty and engage the patient in pelvic floor therapy/biofeedback. If bladder neck reconstruction is performed with the goal of spontaneous voiding, patient/family engagement in behavioral modification and pelvic floor therapy/biofeedback are critical. Notably, bladder capacity may appear low on voiding cystourethrogram or urodynamic studies in individuals who have never had significant bladder outlet resistance. In such cases, the authors find bladder capacity more accurately assessed intraoperatively, where fluid is passively instilled into the bladder under 30 cm H_2O of pressure while bladder outlet resistance is temporarily introduced with an inflated balloon of the urethral Foley catheter occluding the bladder neck. Exstrophy bladders may stretch following introduction of bladder neck resistance and judicious use of beta 3 agonists and/or anticholinergics. Bladder augmentation with aggressive bladder neck reconstruction or bladder neck closure is reserved for those with severely contracted bladders with low compliance or those whose bladder neck anatomy is not amenable for reconstruction.

Omphalocele–exstrophy–imperforate anus–spinal anomalies complex

Given the high prevalence of spinal defects in the OEIS population, voluntary urinary control and detrusor contractions are typically not an option. When patients and parents/caregivers are socially ready, bladder neck closure and continent catheterizable channels are typically created with or without augmentation enterocystoplasty in order to achieve continence. In a study reporting long-term continence outcomes in OEIS complex, 40 of 73 (56%) achieved dryness. Two of the 40 required neobladder. Of the dry patients with intact native bladders, 23 of 38 (84%) required augmentation cystoplasty and 30 of 38 (79%) required a continent catheterizable channel. Only 9 of the 40 (24%) maintained a patent and continent urethra, 6 of which were skin-covered variants. Those with persistent incontinence either had unsuccessful surgeries or were not clinically suited for major urinary reconstruction.[59]

Renal

Proximal epispadias/bladder exstrophy

Baseline renal function is typically normal in patients with epispadias and bladder exstrophy. However, the kidneys are at higher risk of renal scarring from pyelonephritis owing to high prevalence (68%–83%) of vesicoureteral reflux following bladder closure and introduction of resistance at bladder outlet level.[60–62]

Early studies reported poor renal outcomes, particularly in patients who required bladder augmentation or ileal loop conduits, with 10% of deaths attributed to renal failure resulting from recurrent pyelonephritis/renal scarring. Renal function deteriorated in 70% of those who underwent ureterosigmoidostomy. Comparatively, patients that underwent primary bladder closure had less functional deterioration of upper tracts.[63,64]

In a report from Husmann and colleagues,[65] 10 of 68 (15%) of the patients who underwent staged reconstruction developed renal scarring. Gargollo and colleagues[66] reported that 6 of 32 (19%) patients who underwent CPRE had cortical defects on dimercapto succinic acid with median follow-up of 5 years. Notably, 9 of 32 (28%) had 1 to 4 episodes of pyelonephritis. Ellison and colleagues[67] reported renal outcomes in 30 patients following bladder closure with median follow-up of 9.7 years. Mean glomerular filtration rate was normal, although male sex was associated with hydronephrosis and lower glomerular filtration rate. Bilateral ureteral reimplant was performed in 73% of patients for persistent vesicoureteral reflux, recurrent urinary tract infection, and worsening hydronephrosis. More recently, Sinatti and colleagues[68] reported renal outcomes in 48 patients with EEC (15% epispadias, 80% bladder exstrophy, 6% OEIS). Renal function was comparable to age-matched controls with only 2 of 48 (4%) with Society of Fetal Urology grade 2 hydronephrosis. Continence was found to be associated with presence of vesicoureteral reflux.

Omphalocele–exstrophy–imperforate anus–spinal anomalies complex

Patients with OEIS are at particularly high risk for chronic kidney disease owing to baseline dysplasia. Anatomic anomalies of the upper tracts are present in 41% to 66%, including agenesis, dysplasia, fusion, and ectopia.[8,53,69] Following urinary reconstruction, the upper tracts are at risk of damage from high-pressure bladder dynamics, pyelonephritis, and vesicoureteral reflux. Vesicoureteral reflux has been reported in 50% to 60% following reconstruction and may need to be addressed at time of urinary reconstruction.[70] Acute renal dysfunction in pelvic ectopic kidneys is of particular concern during bladder closure owing to an abrupt increase in abdominal/pelvic pressure following pubic bone approximation during second-stage OEIS closure (eg, compartment syndrome).

Sexual

Epispadias

In 2015, 15 adult male patients with epispadias completed a nonvalidated survey on sexual function. Eleven of 15 (73%) reported engaging in sexual intercourse. Eight of 15 (67%) reported decreased ejaculation (n = 6) and anejaculation (n = 2). Four of 15 (27%) reported difficulty with orgasm; 3 of 15 (20%) reported diminished sensation; 3 of 15 (20%) reported difficulty maintaining erection, and 1 of 15 (7%) reported abnormally curved erection. Despite this, 12 of 15 (80%) reported overall satisfaction with sexual intercourse.[71] In a small study of 5 patients, 4 of 5 women with isolated epispadias responded to having good self-confidence and satisfaction in their sexual relationships.[72]

Male bladder exstrophy

Specifically in male exstrophy patients, anatomic anomalies that may impact sexual function include dorsal tethering, dorsal penile curvature, penile torsion owing to corporal disproportion, possible injury to neurovascular bundle during past surgeries, retrograde or anejaculation owing to injury of ejaculatory ducts/bulbospongiosus muscle, and diminished size of phallus.

There is extensive literature reporting sexual health and functioning in male bladder exstrophy patients. In integrated age populations, 71% to 73% reported dating; 58% to 72% reported participating in sexual activity; 84% to 94% reported erections; 22% to 55% reported masturbation; and 59% to 84% reported ejaculation.[73–80] In

adults, 75% to 89% reported sexual activity; greater than 90% reported erections, but 37% to 42% had erections always or often hard enough for penetration; 63% to 69% always or often experienced orgasm; and 32% would feel content or excellent if their current sex life did not change.[81–84]

Female bladder exstrophy

Most adult female exstrophy patients will have some degree of pelvic organ prolapse.[85] Pelvic organ prolapse is due to anterior divergence of pelvic muscles. Furthermore, anterior displacement/horizontal axis of vagina results in cervix uteri that enters the vagina closer to the introitus than typical. Greater than 50% of female patients require surgical correction of vaginal stenosis for sexual intercourse.[86,87]

Female adolescents with bladder exstrophy reported lower scores on all subscales and overall sexual function on the Female Sexual Function Index compared with healthy norms.[80] In adult women, 67% to 84% of women reported experience in sexual activity, and 22% to 42% reported having dyspareunia. Eleven percent of women reported avoidance of sexual intercourse owing to genital prolapse. Thirty-five percent of women reported complete satisfaction with their sexual lives and reached orgasms. Nearly half of sexually active patients reported problems in sexual life owing to incontinence, reduction or lack of clitoral sensitivity, and dyspareunia.[88–91]

Omphalocele–exstrophy–imperforate anus–spinal anomalies complex

Sexual function in individuals affected by OEIS depends on the extent of genital and Mullerian anomalies, which can vary significantly in severity. What further complicated this matter is that, historically, genetically male patients with diminutive phallus not suitable for reconstruction often underwent early orchiectomy and were raised as an individual with female gender. However, cloacal exstrophy male patients typically have normal functioning testicles, thus, normal androgen imprinting in utero. Cloacal exstrophy should not be considered a disorder of sexual differentiation.[59]

Fertility

Case reports and small case series suggest that male patients with bladder exstrophy have oligospermia, azoospermia, asthenospermia, decreased sperm motility, and low ejaculate volumes.[88–92] In one case series, semen analyses from 8 of 25 men with bladder exstrophy showed low ejaculate volume in 6 specimens, normal sperm count in 5, and oligospermia in 3. Normal sperm motility and viability were maintained in half of the specimens.[93] Despite high prevalence of abnormal semen parameters in men with bladder exstrophy, studies have demonstrated that patients can achieve fertility naturally and through assistive reproductive technology.[94]

Female bladder exstrophy appears to also have an impact on female infertility and fetal/neonatal outcome. Case reports and series have described successful pregnancies and delivery in women with bladder exstrophy.[95,96] However, impaired fertility, poor fetal/neonatal outcome, and a risk of significant maternal complications at delivery were reported in a case series of 52 women (mean age, 33 years) with classic bladder exstrophy. Of the women who had tried to become pregnant, approximately two-thirds (19 of 28 patients) were able to conceive. For the 19 women who had conceived, there were a total of 57 pregnancies, including 3 sets of twins. Outcomes of these pregnancies were 34 live births (56%), 21 miscarriages (35%), 4 still births or neonatal deaths, and 1 termination. There were 4 major maternal delivery room complications, including 2 women with postpartum hemorrhage, one patient with transection of the ureter, and one with fistula formation.[86]

Body Image

Several studies based on patient surveys and interviews report that adolescents and young adults with bladder exstrophy are dissatisfied with their genital and body appearance. Their poor body image results in avoidance of undressing or showering in front of others, low rates of masturbation and genital touching, anxiety in establishing a close sexual relationship, and restricting sexual activity.[73,97,98]

Psychological

Studies that used validated survey tools for psychological evaluation report that patients with bladder exstrophy are at risk for anxiety, depression, and adjustment disorder.[74] Results also suggest that incontinence was associated with increased psychological dysfunction.[99] Other reports based on patient interviews or study-designed surveys also demonstrated increased anxiety and need for psychological support.[74,100]

Health-Related Quality of Life

Despite the number of long-term sequelae associated with bladder exstrophy, adolescent patients may adapt to the challenges of their disorder. This was illustrated in a study that surveyed adolescents with bladder exstrophy and epispadias using a validated quality-of-health questionnaire. Although the majority of patients reported incontinence with a median 9 surgical procedures, patients with exstrophy/epispadias had similar scores in nearly all domains compared with those of a normal reference control population.[101]

In a study from a single center that evaluated quality-of-life outcome in children between 8 and 17 years of age, patients with bladder exstrophy had higher health-related quality-of-life scores for physical functioning and overall quality of life compared with children with kidney stones and the general pediatric population. These surprising findings were attributed to the aggressive and comprehensive medical, surgical, and psychosocial care provided to this cohort of patients with bladder exstrophy. However, patients with bladder exstrophy with lower scores for body image were more likely to have lower social and emotional function scores and less likely to have romantic relationships.[102]

The above-mentioned results must be interpreted with caution. Existing generic health-related quality-of-life instruments may not accurately capture how manifestations of the disease (ie, incontinence, sexual dysfunction, poor body image) truly impact quality of life. Condition-specific surveys and instruments for ECC, which have not yet been developed, may be valuable tools in understanding the health-related quality of life of patients affected by EEC.

SUMMARY

Each entity within the EEC spectrum presents with a unique set of pathologic conditions that must be approached with care and caution. Timely diagnosis and appropriate counseling during the perinatal period are imperative. Reconstruction should be performed by an experienced surgeon and team familiar with the intricacies of EEC anatomy and sequelae of major reconstruction. Regardless of initial surgical approach, patients affected by EEC frequently struggle with long-term incontinence and sexual dysfunction that need to be addressed through an individualized approach, taking into consideration both psychosocial and anatomic factors.

CLINICS CARE POINTS

Epispadias

- Although there is higher likelihood of continence for individuals with more distal meatal location, there is still a significant portion of patients with distal meatal location that struggle with life-long incontinence.

- Depending on baseline continence status and appearance of the bladder neck, surgical management ranges from isolated penile repair to concomitant bladder neck reconstruction, with or without pelvic bone osteotomies.

Bladder Exstrophy

- Regardless of technique, the rate of complete continence through voluntary voiding is quite low following initial surgery.

- Additional surgeries, including bladder neck reconstruction, bladder neck closure, augmentation cystoplasty, and/or continent catheterizable channels, are required to improve continence.

- Management of persistent continence should be highly individualized depending on each patient's anatomy and psychosocial situation.

Omphalocele–Exstrophy–Imperforate Anus–Spinal Anomalies Complex

- Patients with omphalocele–exstrophy–imperforate anus–spinal anomalies complex are at particularly high risk for chronic kidney disease owing to baseline anatomic anomalies of the upper tracts and congenital renal dysplasia.

- The initial goal of genitourinary reconstruction is to bring the 2 hemibladder plates together by excising the omphalocele and separating the cecal plate from bladder halves.

- The second stage of the procedure is similar to reconstruction of bladder exstrophy, with steps including iliac osteotomies, bladder closure, urethroplasty, and reconstruction of external genitalia.

- Given the high prevalence of spinal defects in the omphalocele–exstrophy-imperforate anus–spinal anomalies complex population, voluntary urinary control and detrusor contractions are typically not an option. When patients and parents/caregivers are socially ready, bladder neck closure and continent catheterizable channels are typically created with or without augmentation enterocystoplasty in order to achieve continence.

REFERENCES

1. Anonymous. Epidemiology of bladder exstrophy and epispadias: a communication from the International Clearinghouse for Birth Defects Monitoring Systems. Teratology 1987;36:221–7.

2. Gambhir L, Höller T, Müller M, et al. Epidemiological survey of 214 European families with Bladder Exstrophy-Epispadias Complex (BEEC). J Urol 2008;179(4):1539–43.

3. Allen L, Rodjani A, Kelly J, et al. Female epispadias: are we missing the diagnosis. BJU Int 2004; 94:613–5.

4. Yang P, Khoury MJ, Stewart WF, et al. Comparative epidemiology of selected midline congenital abnormalities. Genet Epidemiol 1994;11:141–54.

5. Martinez-Frias ML, Bermejo E, Rodriguez-Pinilla E, et al. Exstrophy of the cloaca and exstrophy of the bladder: two different expressions of a primary developmental field defect. Am J Med Genet 2001;99:261–9.

6. Nelson CP, Dunn RL, Wei JT. Contemporary epidemiology of bladder exstrophy in the United States. J Urol 2005;173:1728–31.

7. Caton AR, Bloom A, Druschel CM, et al. Epidemiology of bladder and cloacal exstrophies in New York State, 1983- 1999. Birth Defects Res A Clin Mol Teratol 2007;79:781–7.

8. Hurwitz RS, Manzoni GA, Ransley PG, et al. Cloacal exstrophy: a report of 34 cases. J Urol 1987;138:1060–4.

9. Moore CA, Weaver DD. Exstrophy of cloaca sequence. In: Buyse ML, editor. Birth defects encyclopedia. Dover (MA): Centers for Birth defects Information Services, Inc; 1990. p. 648–9.

10. Boyadjiev SA, Dodson JL, Radford CL, et al. Clinical and molecular characterization of the bladder exstrophy-epispadias complex: analysis of 232 families. BJU Int 2004;94:1337–43.

11. Muecke EC. The role of the cloacal membrane in exstrophy: the first successful experimental study. J Urol 1964;92:659–67.

12. Austin PF, Homsy YL, Gearhart JP, et al. Prenatal diagnosis of cloacal exstrophy. J Urol 1998;160: 1179–81.

13. Van der Putte SC. Normal and abnormal development of the anorectum. J Pediatr Surg 1986;21: 434–40.

14. Thomalla JV, Rudolph RA, Rink RC, et al. Induction of cloacal exstrophy in the chick embryo using the CO_2 laser. J Urol 1985;134:991–5.

15. Beaudoin S, Simon L, Bargy F. Anatomical basis of the common embryological origin for epispadias and bladder or cloacal exstrophy. Surg Radiol Anat 1997;19:11–6.

16. Beaudoin S, Barbet P, Bargy F. Pelvic development in the rabbit embryo: implications in the organogenesis of bladder exstrophy. Anat Embryol 2004; 208:425–30.

17. Ambrose SS, O'Brien DP. Surgical embryology of the exstrophy-epispadias complex. Surg Clin North Am 1974;54:1379.

18. Johnston JH, Kogan SJ. The exstrophic anomalies and their surgical reconstruction. Curr Probl Surg 1974;46:1–39.

19. Mildenberger H, Lkuth D, Dziuba M. Embryology of bladder exstrophy. J Pediatr Surg 1988;23:116.

20. Gondo K, Yokomine M, Yoshizato T, et al. Clues and pitfalls in prenatal diagnosis of classic cloacal exstrophy using ultrasonography and magnetic resonance imaging: A case with sequential observation from 17 to 30 weeks' gestation and literature review. J Obstet Gynaecol Res 2020;46:1443–9.

21. Weiss DA, Oliver ER, Borer JG, et al. Key anatomic findings on fetal ultrasound and MRI in the prenatal diagnosis of bladder and cloacal exstrophy. J Pediatr Urol 2020;16(5):665–71.

22. Gearhart JP, Ben-Chaim J, Jeffs RD, et al. Criteria for the prenatal diagnosis of classic bladder exstrophy. Obstet Gynecol 1995;85:961–4.

23. Lee T, Weiss D, Roth E, et al. Prenatal Diagnosis of Bladder Exstrophy and OEIS over 20 Years. Urology 2022;172:174–7.

24. Sponseller PD, Bisson LJ, Gearhart JP, et al. The anatomy of the pelvis in the exstrophy complex. J Bone Joint Surg Am 1995;77:177–89.

25. Stec AA. Embryology and bony and pelvic floor anatomy in the bladder exstrophy epispadias complex. Semin Pediatr Surg 2011;20:66–70.

26. Ransley PG, Duffy PG, Wollin M. Bladder exstrophyclosure and epispadias repair. In: Ransley PG, Duffy PG, Wollin M, editors. Operative surgery-PediatricSurgery. 4th edition. London: Butterworths; 1989. p. 620.

27. Mitchell ME, Bagli DJ. Complete penile disassembly for epispadias repair: the Mitchell technique. J Urol 1996;155:300.

28. Hernandez DJ, Purves T, Gearhart JP. Complications of surgical reconstruction of the exstrophy–epispadias complex. J Pediatr Urol 2008;4(6):460–6.

29. Baird AD, Gearhart JP, Mathews RI. Applications of the modified CantwelleRansley epispadias repair in the exstrophy epispadias complex. J Pediatr Urol 2005;1:331e6.

30. Zaontz MR, Steckler RE, Shortliffe LM, et al. Multicenter experience with the Mitchell technique for epispadias repair. J Urol 1998;160:172e6.

31. Gearhart JP, Jeffs RD. State-of-the-art reconstructive surgery for bladder exstrophy at the Johns Hopkins Hospital. Am J Dis Child 1989;143:1475.

32. Jeffs RD, Charrios R, Mnay M, et al. Primary closure of the exstrophied bladder. In: Scott R, editor. Current Controversies in Urologic management. Philadelphia: WB Saunders; 1972. p. 235.

33. Grady RW, Mitchell ME. Newborn exstrophy closure and epispadias repair. World J Urol 1998;16:200.

34. Kelly JH. Vesical exstrophy: repair using radical mobilisation of soft tissues. Pediatr Surg Int 1995;10(5):298–304.

35. Schaeffer AJ, Johnson EK, Logvinenko T, et al. Practice patterns and resource utilization for infants with bladder exstrophy: a national perspective. J Urol 2014;191(5):1381–8.

36. Ahn JJ, Shnorhavorian M, Katz C, et al. Early versus delayed closure of bladder exstrophy: a national surgical quality improvement program pediatric analysis. J Pediatr Urol 2018;14(1):27-e1.

37. Wu WJ, Maruf M, Manyevitch R, et al. Delaying primary closure of classic bladder exstrophy: When is it too late? J Pediatr Urol 2020;16(6):834-e1.

38. Borer JG, Vasquez E, Canning DA, et al. Short-term outcomes of the multi-institutional bladder exstrophy consortium: successes and complications in the first two years of collaboration. J Pediatr Urol 2017;13:275.e1-6, 11. Ferrara F, Dickson AP.

39. Ferrara F, Dickson AP, Fishwick J, et al. Delayed exstrophy repair (DER) does not compromise initial bladder development. J Pediatr Urol 2014;10(3):506–10.

40. Haffar A, Manyevitch R, Morrill C, et al. A Single Center's Changing Trends in the Management and Outcomes of Primary Closure of Classic Bladder Exstrophy: An Evolving Landscape. Urology 2023. https://doi.org/10.1016/j.urology.2022.12.064.

41. Centers of Excellence" Association for the Bladder Exstrophy Community. Available at: https://www.bladderexstrophy.com/centers-excellence/. Accessed April 3, 2023.

42. Papavramidis TS, Marinis AD, Pliakos I, et al. Abdominal compartment syndrome–Intra-abdominal hypertension: Defining, diagnosing, and managing. J Emerg Trauma Shock 2011;4(2):279.

43. Cervellione RM, Husmann DA, Bivalacqua TJ, et al. Penile ischemic injury in the exstrophy/epispadias spectrum: new insights and possible mechanisms. J Pediatr Urol 2010;6(5):450–6.

44. Lloyd JC, Spano SM, Ross SS, et al. How dry is dry? A review of definitions of continence in the contemporary exstrophy/epispadias literature. J Urol 2012;188:1900.

45. Shnorhavorian M, Grady RW, Andersen A, et al. Long-term followup of complete primary repair of exstrophy: the Seattle experience. J Urol 2008;180:1615.

46. Canalichio KL, Ahn J, Hwang C, et al. Long-term urological and gynecological outcomes following complete primary repair in females with bladder exstrophy. J Pediatr Urol 2021;17(5):608-e1.

47. Kramer SA, Kelalis PP. Assessment of Urinary Continence in Epispadias: Review of 94 Patients. J Urol 1982;128:290–3.

48. Mollard P, Basset T, Mure PY. Male Epispadias: Experience with 45 Cases. J Urol 1998;160:55–9.

49. Braga LHP, Lorenzo AJ, Bägli DJ, et al. Outcome Analysis of Isolated Male Epispadias: Single Center Experience With 33 Cases. J Urol 2008;179:1107–12.

50. Thomas JS, Shenoy M, Mushtaq I, et al. Long-term outcomes in primary male epispadias. J Pediatr Urol 2020;16:80.e1-6.

51. Purves JT, Baird AD, Gearhart JP. The modern staged repair of bladder exstrophy in the female: a contemporary series. J Pediatr Urol 2008;4(2):150–3.

52. Cheikhelard A, Aigrain Y, Lottmann H, et al. Female epispadias management: perineal urethrocervicoplasty versus classical Young-Dees procedure. J Urol 2009;182(4):1807–12.

53. Suson KD, Preece J, Baradaran N, et al. The Fate of the Complete Female Epispadias and Exstrophy Bladder—Is There a Difference? J Urol 2013;190(4):1583–9.

54. Maruf M, Manyevitch R, Michaud J, et al. Urinary continence outcomes in classic bladder exstrophy: a long-term perspective. J Urol 2020;203(1):200–5.

55. Ellison JS, Shnorhavorian M, Willihnganz-Lawson K, et al. A critical appraisal of continence in bladder exstrophy: long-term outcomes of the complete primary repair. J Pediatr Urol 2016;12(4):205-e1.

56. Jarzebowski AC, McMullin ND, Grover SR, et al. The Kelly technique of bladder exstrophy repair: continence, cosmesis and pelvic organ prolapse outcome. J Urol 2009;182(4 Suppl):1802–6.

57. Szymanski KM, Fuchs M, Mcleod D, et al. Probability of bladder augmentation, diversion and clean intermittent catheterization in classic bladder exstrophy: a 36-year, multi-institutional, retrospective cohort study. J Urol 2019;202(6):1256–62.

58. Mouriquand PDE, Bubanj T, Feyaerts A, et al. Long-term results of bladder neck reconstruction for incontinence in children with classical bladder exstrophy or incontinent epispadias. BJU Int 2003;92(9):997–1002.

59. Phillips TM, Salmasi AH, Stec A, et al. Urological outcomes in the omphalocele exstrophy imperforate anus spinal defects (OEIS) complex: Experience with 80 patients. J Pediatr Urol 2013;9(3):353–8.

60. Braga LH, Lorenzo AJ, Jrearz R, et al. Bilateral ureteral reimplantation at primary bladder exstrophy closure. J Urol 2010;183(6):2337–41.

61. Ramji J, Weiss DA, Romao RLP, et al. Impact of bilateral ureteral reimplantation at the time of complete primary repair of bladder exstrophy on reflux rates, renogram abnormalities and bladder capacity. J Pediatr Urol 2021;17(3):393.e1.

62. Jarosz SL, Weaver JK, Weiss DA, et al. Bilateral ureteral reimplantation at complete primary repair of exstrophy: Post-operative outcomes. J Pediatr Urol 2022;18(1):37.e1.

63. Turner WR, Ransley PG, Williams DI. Patterns of renal damage in the management of vesical exstrophy. J Urol 1980;124(3):412–5.

64. Mesrobian HG, Kelalis PP, Kramer SA. Long-term followup of 103 patients with bladder exstrophy. J Urol 1988;139:719.

65. Husmann DA, McLorie GA, Churchill BM. Factors predisposing to renal scarring: following staged reconstruction of classical bladder exstrophy. J Pediatr Surg 1990;25(5):500–4.

66. Gargollo PC, Borer JG, Diamond DA, et al. Prospective followup in patients after complete primary repair of bladder exstrophy. J Urol 2008;180(4S):1665–70.

67. Ellison JS, Ahn J, Shnorhavorian M, et al. Long-term fate of the upper tracts following complete primary repair of bladder exstrophy. J Pediatr Urol 2017;13(4):394.e1.

68. Sinatti C, Spinoit AF, Raes A, et al. Long-Term fate of the upper urinary tract and ITS association with continence in exstrophy patients. J Pediatr Urol 2021;17(5):655.e1.

69. Diamond DA. Management of cloacal exstrophy. Dial PediatrUrol 1990;13:2.

70. Stolar CH, Randolph JG, Flanigan LP. Cloacal exstrophy: individualized management through a staged surgical approach. J Pediatr Surg 1990;25(5):505e7.

71. Reddy SS, Inouye BM, Anele UA, et al. Sexual health outcomes in adults with complete male epispadias. J Urol 2015;194(4):1091–5.

72. Amesty MV, Chocarro G, Lobato R, et al. Quality of life in female epispadias. Eur J Pediatr Surg 2016;26(03):277–81.

73. Diseth TH, Bjordal R, Schultz A, et al. Somatic function, mental health and psychosocial functioning in 22 adolescents with bladder exstrophy and epispadias. J Urol 1998;159(5):1684–90.

74. Ebert A, Scheuering S, Schott G, et al. Psychosocial and psychosexual development in childhood and adolescence within the exstrophy-epispadias complex. J Urol 2005;174(3):1094–8.

75. Wilson C, Christie D, Woodhouse CR. The ambitions of adolescents born with exstrophy: a structured survey. BJU Int 2004;94(4):607–12.

76. Jochault-Ritz S, Mercier M, Aubert D. Short and long-term quality of life after reconstruction of bladder exstrophy in infancy: preliminary results of the QUALEX (QUAlity of Life of bladder EXstrophy) study. J Pediatr Surg 2010;45(8):1693–700.

77. Lee C, Reutter HM, GRÄßER MF, et al. Gender-associated differences in the psychosocial and developmental outcome in patients affected with the bladder exstrophy-epispadias complex. BJU Int 2006;97(2):349–53.

78. da Cruz JAS, de Mattos B, Srougi M, et al. Quality of life in young adult patients treated for bladder exstrophy. Cent Eur J Urol 2016;69(2):221.

79. Van Grunsven EJ, Froeling FM, De Vries JD. Outcome analysis of the psychosexual and

socioeconomical development of adult patients born with bladder exstrophy. J Urol 1994;152(5): 1417–9.

80. Deans R, Liao LM, Wood D, et al. Sexual function and health-related quality of life in women with classic bladder exstrophy. BJU Int 2015;115(4): 633–8.

81. Bujons A, Lopategui DM, Rodríguez N, et al. Quality of life in female patients with bladder exstrophy-epispadias complex: Long-term follow-up. J Pediatr Urol 2016;12(4):210-e1.

82. Traceviciute J, Zwink N, Jenetzky E, et al. Sexual function and quality of life in adult male individuals with exstrophy-epispadias complex—A survey of the German CURE-Network. Urology 2018;112: 215–21.

83. Catti M, Paccalin C, Rudigoz RC, et al. Quality of life for adult women born with bladder and cloacal exstrophy: a long-term follow up. J Pediatr Urol 2006;2(1):16–22.

84. Gupta AD, Goel SK, Woodhouse CR, et al. Examining long-term outcomes of bladder exstrophy: a 20-year follow-up. BJU Int 2014;113(1):137–41.

85. Kaufman MR. Pelvic organ prolapse and pregnancy in the female bladder exstrophy patient. Curr Urol Rep 2018;19:1–7.

86. Woodhouse CRJ, Hinsch R. The anatomy and reconstruction of the adult female genitalia in classical exstrophy. Br J Urol 1997;79(4):618–22.

87. Cervellione RM, Phillips T, Baradaran N, et al. Vaginoplasty in the female exstrophy population: Outcomes and complications. J Pediatr Urol 2010; 6(6):595–9.

88. Tank ES, Lindenauer SM. Principles of management of exstrophy of the cloaca. Am J Surg 1970; 119(1):95–8.

89. Stein R, Stöckle M, Fisch M, et al. The fate of the adult exstrophy patient. J Urol 1994;152:1413.

90. Ben-Chaim J, Jeffs RD, Reiner WG, et al. The outcome of patients with classic bladder exstrophy in adult life. J Urol 1996;155:1251.

91. Mesrobian HG, Kelalis PP, Kramer SA. Long-term followup of cosmetic appearance and genital function in boys with exstrophy: review of 53 patients. J Urol 1986;136:256.

92. Lattimer JK, MacFarlane MT, Puchner PJ. Male exstrophy patients: a preliminary report on the reproductive capability. Trans Am Assoc Genitourin Surg 1978;70:42.

93. Hanna MK, Williams DI. Genital function in males with vesical exstrophy and epispadias. Br J Urol 1972;44:169.

94. Avolio L, Koo HP, Bescript AC, et al. The long-term outcome in men with exstrophy/epispadias: sexual function and social integration. J Urol 1996;156: 822.

95. Reynaud N, Courtois F, Mouriquand P, et al. Male sexuality, fertility, and urinary continence in bladder exstrophy-epispadias complex. J Sex Med 2018; 15(3):314–23.

96. Mathews RI, Gan M, Gearhart JP. Urogynaecological and obstetric issues in women with the exstrophy-epispadias complex. BJU Int 2003;91: 845.

97. Deans R, Banks F, Liao LM, et al. Reproductive outcomes in women with classic bladder exstrophy: an observational cross-sectional study. Am J Obstet Gynecol 2012;206:496.e1.

98. Reiner WG, Gearhart JP, Jeffs R. Psychosexual dysfunction in males with genital anomalies: late adolescence, Tanner stages IV to VI. J Am Acad Child Adolesc Psychiatry 1999;38:865.

99. Diseth TH, Emblem R, Schultz A. Mental health, psychosocial functioning, and quality of life in patients with bladder exstrophy and epispadias - an overview. World J Urol 1999;17:239.

100. Reiner WG, Gearhart JP. Anxiety disorders in children with epispadias-exstrophy. Urology 2006;68: 172.

101. Schaeffer AJ, Yenokyan G, Alcorn K, et al. Health related quality of life in adolescents with bladder exstrophy-epispadias as measured by the Child Health Questionnaire-Child Form 87. J Urol 2012; 188:1924.

102. Pennison MC, Mednick L, Rosoklija I, et al. Health related quality of life in patients with bladder exstrophy: a call for targeted interventions. J Urol 2014; 191:1553.

Neurogenic Lower Urinary Tract Dysfunction

John S. Wiener, MD[a],*, Rajeev Chaudhry, MD[b]

KEYWORDS

- Neurogenic bladder • Neuropathic bladder • Diseases • Urinary tract • Spina bifida
- Urinary incontinence • Diagnostic techniques • Urological

KEY POINTS

- NLUTD in children is typically congenital and most commonly due to spina bifida but can present across a wide spectrum of bladder and renal dysfunction.
- Guidleines for management of NLUTD are well-defined and provide great diagnostic and therapeutic detail; they do skew towards proactive management.
- The need for intervention is guided by potential or actual renal damage, history of recurrent UTI, and desire for urinary continence and/or independence.

Neurogenic lower urinary tract dysfunction (NLUTD), although not common in the general population, can account for a significant portion of the practice of pediatric urologists. Unlike many other pediatric urologic disorders which are primarily treated to improve quality of life (QOL)—often far in the future, NLUTD must be appropriately managed, often beginning at birth, to prevent or minimize complications of urinary tract infection (UTI) and chronic kidney disease (CKD) which can seriously affect a child's health in the near term in addition to impaired bladder and bowel function which can negatively affect QOL. Most of the children with NLUTD require regular surveillance throughout childhood and adulthood, and a few will need to undergo some of the most complex surgeries performed by pediatric urologists.[1]

CAUSES

NLUTD is defined by bladder and/or sphincteric dysfunction caused by a neuropathy (**Box 1**). The neuropathy can be congenital or acquired, can be central or peripheral, and can be permanent or transient. Approaching NLUTD in children can be fundamentally different than in adults because most cases are congenital; thus, affected nerves and the genitourinary tract may malformed and dysfunctional before birth, limiting the ability to achieve more normal function and morphology.

The most common cause of congenital NLUTD is neural tube defects. Spina bifida (SB) is the most common nonchromosomal birth defect affecting multiple organ systems with an incidence of 3.1 per 10,000 births in the United States (US).[2] About 1400 children are born with SB each year in the United States with Hispanic children having the highest incidence.[3] Maternal folic acid deficiency or impairment of folate-mediated metabolism can result in improper closure of the neural tube during embryonic life. To combat this, US governmental agencies recommended that all women of childbearing age consume 400 mcg of folic acid daily and mandated enrichment of all processed grains with folic acid; this led to a 24% reduction in the occurrence of SB.[4] Myelomeningocele is the most severe form of SB, and NLUTD is expected.[5] Data from the National Spina Bifida Patient Registry found only 20%, 15%, and 10% of school-aged, adolescent, and adult patients, respectively, managed their bladders by volitional voiding, and those with myelomeningocele had greater dysfunction.[6]

[a] Department of Urology, Duke University Medical Center, Box 3831, Durham, NC 27710, USA; [b] University of Pittsburgh Medical Center, Children's Hospital of Pittsburgh, 4401 Penn Avenue, Pittsburgh, PA 15224, USA
* Corresponding author.
E-mail address: john.wiener@duke.edu

Urol Clin N Am 50 (2023) 415–432
https://doi.org/10.1016/j.ucl.2023.04.002
0094-0143/23/© 2023 Elsevier Inc. All rights reserved.

Box 1
Causes of neurogenic lower urinary tract dysfunction

Congenital

  Spina bifida (neural tube defect)

    Myelomeningocele

    Lipomyelomeningocele

    Meningocele

    Split cord malformation

    Terminal myelocystocele

    Tethered cord

  Sacral agenesis

  Sacrococcygeal teratoma

  Anorectal malformations

  Brain conditions: cerebral palsy, brain malformations

Acquired

  Spinal cord injury: traumatic/iatrogenic

  Secondary spinal cord tethering after previous surgery

  Transverse myelitis

  Peripheral nerve injury during pelvic surgery[a]

  Brain conditions: brain injury, tumors, encephalopathies

[a]Peripherial nerves can be injured during pelvic surgery for resection of sacrococcygeal teratomas and other pelvic malignancies, correction of anorectal malformations, and correction of bladder/bilateral ureteral conditions (vesicoureteral reflux).

Other causes of congenital NLUTD include sacral agenesis, anorectal malformations, and sacrococcygeal teratoma. The neuropathy of the latter two may be due to congenital malformation of bladder and sphincteric nerves in the pelvis or secondary to iatrogenic injury when surgery is performed to manage these problems. Sacral agenesis is more similar to neural tube defects with abnormal neural function before birth and is more common in offspring of diabetic mothers.[7] Congenital or birth-related brain malformations and trauma can also cause NLUTD.

Acquired NLUTD can result from spinal cord injury (SCI) which may be traumatic or iatrogenic during spinal surgery. Delayed neuropathy can occur from secondary spinal cord tethering related to scarring from prior cord surgery, such as initial SB back closure. Rarer forms of spinal cord pathology include transverse myelitis, spinal cord infarction, and tumors. Brain injury, tumors, and encephalitis can cause central nerve system-mediated NLUTD. Finally, peripheral nerve injury, most likely, during pelvic surgery, is a rare etiology of NLUTD in children.

NATURAL HISTORY

Before the modern era, NLUTD often resulted in significant morbidity and mortality. Our improved understanding of normal and altered bladder function has allowed most children with NLUTD to survive childhood, rather than succumb to uropathies, such as pyelonephritis and CKD. Like all disorders, NLUTD occurs as a spectrum, from mild voiding symptoms to hostile bladder leading to end-stage renal failure. Children, unlike adults, are dynamic beings, and alterations in neurologic function leading to progression of NLUTD can occur during normal childhood and pubertal growth.

NLUTD can simply be categorized as failure of the bladder to store and/or to empty urine. Failure to store urine can result from sphincteric inadequacy and/or bladder characteristics that increase bladder pressure, forcing urine out involuntarily. Failure to empty may be a consequence of failure of the bladder outlet's to open properly and/or the bladder detrusor muscle to contract in an organized and sustained manner to properly evacuate the bladder. Central nervous system pathology may cause NLUTD due to improper initiation or coordination of the bladder and bladder outlet during voiding.

NLUTD may result in failure to toilet train or cause new onset of incontinence in older children. Although this may degrade QOL, other potential consequences are more ominous. Inadequate emptying and/or excessive bladder storage pressures can increase the risk of UTI. Before reliable antibiotics and modern management strategies, UTIs could be fatal. CKD and renal failure are the most feared complications of NLUTD today as renal deterioration can be silent but progressive—a result of excessive bladder storage pressures. High pressure in the bladder can prevent the ureters from emptying and/or force urine to reflux up the ureters, either resulting in increased pressure in the upper tracts or promoting pyelonephritis, both of which can destroy nephrons. Urinary diversion procedures were common in such children in the past to arrest this progression.[8] The past 50 years have seen the advent of clean intermittent catheterization (CIC) to reliably empty the bladder as well as medical and surgical interventions to reduce bladder storage pressure and improve continence, allowing most children with severe NLUTD to avoid urinary diversion and enjoy longer and happier lives.[9]

GOALS OF MANAGEMENT

The goals of management of NLUTD are (1) protection of renal function, (2) minimizing UTI, (3) attainment of continence, and (4) achievement of independence during the transition to adulthood. Most children with congenital NLUTD, specifically SB, are born with normal kidneys.[10] The pediatric urologist's job is to ensure that the child grows up with normal renal function and maintains that when fully grown to avoid CKD. It may not be possible to completely prevent UTI, but minimizing their occurrence can reduce morbidity and better preserve renal parenchyma. Most children with NLUTD can achieve urinary continence with stepwise management moving from behavioral to medical to surgical interventions, depending on the type and severity of NLUTD. Not all patients are willing to take the necessary steps for continence or have the social support to ensure compliance, so the goal of continence is more subjective than the first two goals. As survival into adulthood is becoming the norm for most of these children, helping the adolescent move from dependence on parents and caregivers to being able to manage their bladder independently is a critical issue.[11] Optimization of bowel and sexual dysfunction that may accompany NLUTD cannot be ignored and can improve urinary function, but these topics are beyond the scope of this article.

GUIDELINES

Multiple guidelines exist for management of NLUTD (**Table 1**). They are skewed heavily toward SB because of its preponderance of cases of pediatric NLUTD. In 2018, the Spina Bifida Association produced its fourth edition of Guidelines for the Care of People Living with Spina Bifida, and the urology chapter provides an age-based protocol for management with a list of research gaps.[12,13] The European Association of Urology has a section on Management of Neurogenic Bladder in its 2022 Guidelines on Pediatric Urology.[14] The British Association of Pediatric Urologists published a consensus statement on the management of neuropathic bladder (synonymous with neurogenic bladder or NLUTD) in 2016.[15] Finally, the International Children's Continence Society produced recommendations for initial workup and subsequent follow-up of neuropathic bladder in 2012.[16]

Consideration of these guidelines necessitates an understanding of the evolution of management of pediatric NLUTD. Before the late twentieth century, physicians reactively treated NLUTD after clinical evidence of morbidity in the form of upper urinary tract damage, recurrent UTI, or persistent incontinence. Incontinent urinary diversion to an external appliance or cutaneous vesicostomy was commonplace and preferable to the constant care and complications of suprapubic bladder catheters.[7] The introduction of the concept of CIC and pharmacotherapy to reduce detrusor muscle uninhibited contractions (neurogenic detrusor overactivity [NDO]) and/or elevated tone allowed urologists to reactively treat patients nonsurgically,[17,18] and bladder augmentation procedures made possible continent reconstructive options in those who failed medical therapy. However, these forms of management were performed after NLUTD was noted to progress in children; this approach is called *reactive* or *expectant*. The alternative approach which has gained popularity over the past 40 years is *proactive* management of NLUTD.[19] Proactive management can refer to (1) either universal initiation of medical management with CIC and/or anticholinergic medication in all children with NLUTD beginning at birth or diagnosis or (2) early urodynamic evaluation to assess bladder hostility and intervention for those demonstrating features predictive of upper tract deterioration. This proactive approach is widely practiced today with two of the four guidelines in **Table 1**, labeling themselves as proactive (European Association of Urology [EAU] and International Children's Continence Society [ICCS]), a third (Spina Bifida Association [SBA]) combining aspects of both proactive and reactive management, and the fourth not taking a side as it was a survey rather than a recommendation. Although the proactive approach may seem intuitive, it can create morbidity associated with CIC or anticholinergic medication as well as unnecessary costs and burden on caregivers, and some argue that it does not improve long-term outcomes.[20]

IMAGING

As the primary goal of management is to protect the kidneys, imaging is central to the management of NLUTD. For expectant management, upper tract changes are the impetus to modify therapy, but even with good proactive management, unanticipated changes can occur. It is thought that an early detection of upper tract changes allows for intervention before changes are permanent and lead to CKD.[19] Therefore, imaging must be performed regularly with some degree of uniformity among the various guidelines. It is important to have a historic perspective because before the late twentieth century, radiographic monitoring meant periodic intravenous pyelograms (IVP) with its downsides of cumulative radiation dosing along

Table 1
Current guidelines for management of pediatric neurogenic lower urinary tract dysfunction

	SBA Guidelines[12,13]	EAU Guidelines[14]	BAPU Consensus Statement[15]	ICCS Recommendations[16]
General approach	"... merges aspects of proactive & reactive philosophies based on a best practices methodology"	Proactive	Not applicable in this survey of practice preferences	Proactive
Renal bladder US	• After birth • At 6, 12, 18, and 24 mo • Repeat annually • Repeat if symptomatic UTI or worsening urodynamics develop	• After birth • Repeat annually	• Part of initial assessment • For stable bladder on CIC, should be performed at least yearly	• Part of initial evaluation • At 6, 12, 18, and 24 mo in those with NDO • Yearly or biannually after toddler; resume yearly in adolescence, then biannually after growth spurt to triannually in adulthood
Laboratory evaluation	• Serum creatinine in first 3 mo of life • Repeat if upper tract changes noted • Repeat at age 5 y and then annually • Consider alternative measure of renal function if low muscle mass	• Serum creatinine in first week of life • "Lifelong follow-up of renal function" • Serum cystatin C may be more accurate later in life	No consensus	• Serum creatinine after first week of life, if indicated • Follow-up not addressed
DMSA scan	No recommendation	Obtain baseline in first year of life	Not performed unless clinical or radiological indications develop	• Consider if VUR or renal scarring noted • Repeat if numerous febrile UTI occur

Urodynamics			
• Initial study in first 3 mo • Repeat annually until age 3 y • Repeat if patient has recurrent UTI, upper tract changes, or desire for/changes in continence	• Initial study in first 2–3 mo • Repeat annually depending on clinical situation • Fluoroscopy or VCUG may be helpful	• In newborn, it "is reasonable… on a select few, based on clinical and radiological assessment" • For stable bladder on CIC can be reserved for clinical or radiological indications	• Initial study after child stabilized postoperatively for open SB • Initial study before spinal cord detethering surgery for closed SB • At least 6 wk (preferably 3 mo) after SCI • Repeat yearly during toddler years, then later only if US shows change in residual urine, hydronephrosis, or bladder wall thickening; after recurrent UTI; or change noted in continence or lower extremity function • Repeat 2–3 mo after initiation of anticholinergic medication when indicated • VCUG recommended if hydronephrosis, ureteral dilation, discrepancy in renal sizes/contour, increased bladder wall thickness noted or UDS reveal NDO, poor compliance, elevated LPP or DSD • Repeat VCUG if VUR, upper tract dilation, poor renal growth, loss of parenchyma, or symptomatic pyelonephritis noted

(continued on next page)

Table 1
(continued)

	SBA Guidelines[12,13]	EAU Guidelines[14]	BAPU Consensus Statement[15]	ICCS Recommendations[16]
Clean intermittent catheterization (CIC)	• Initiate for mixed incontinence when indicated by upper tract changes, recurrent symptomatic UTI, or bladder hostility noted on UDS • Involve child in process beginning at age 3–5 y	• Early initiation suggested • Can delay if underactive sphincter or no DSD noted	• No consensus to use universally vs only in select patients	• At diagnosis, perform until UDS is done if child is not emptying bladder spontaneously • Perform in cases with high grade VUR or NDO along with starting anticholinergic medication • Initiate as soon as feasible after SCI
Anticholinergic medication	• Initiate for mixed incontinence when indicated by upper tract changes, recurrent symptomatic UTI, or bladder hostility noted on UDS	• Initiate early (in newborns) if suspicion of NDO • Use botulinum toxin if refractory • Bladder augmentation surgery recommended if poor response	• No consensus on routine use • Oxybutynin is first-line agent • Reasonable to use botulinum toxin to improve compliance • Bladder augmentation with ileum preferred when indicated	• Use in cases with high-grade VUR or NDO along with starting CIC • Use in cases with high filling pressures
Incontinence	• Discuss urinary continence program at each visit beginning at age 6 y • No surgical recommendations given	• Offer bladder outlet surgery if sphincter weak • Combine with bladder augmentation in most patients	Not addressed	Not addressed
Continent catheterizable channel	Not addressed	• Offer in patients with difficulty catheterizing per urethra	Not addressed	Not addressed
Urinary tract infections	• Specific definitions given • Treat only if definitions met • Catheterized specimen encouraged	Treat only if symptomatic	Not addressed	Not addressed

Vitamin B12 and serum chemistries	Lifelong follow-up if ileum used for reconstructive surgery	Check yearly beginning 2 y after reconstructive surgery	Not addressed	Not addressed
Cystoscopy	In adults after bladder augmentation only if upper tract changes, gross hematuria, symptomatic UTI, worsening incontinence, pelvic pain, or renal transplant with BK/polyoma virus noted	Consider annually beginning 10–15 y after reconstructive surgery	Not indicated in first 10 y after bladder augmentation except in immune-compromised or symptomatic patients	Not addressed
Transition to self-management	Begin at age 13–17 y.	Not addressed	Not addressed	Not addressed
Bowel management	• Discuss bowel management program at each visit beginning at 3 y • See separate guidelines	Recommend program to achieve continence and independence	Not addressed	Should be evaluated and treated appropriately
Sexuality	• See separate guidelines	Initiate discussion in adolescence	Not addressed	Not addressed

Abbreviations: BAPU, British Association of Paediatric Urologists; CIC, clean intermittent catheterization; DMSA, dimercaptosuccinic acid nuclear renal scan; DSD, detrusor sphincter dyssynergia; EAU, European Association of Urology; ICCS, International Children's Continence Society; LPP, leak point pressure; NDO, neurogenic detrusor overactivity; SB, spina bifida; SBA, Spina Bifida Association; SCI, spinal cord injury; UDS, urodynamic study; US, ultrasound; UTI, urinary tract infection(s); VCUG, voiding cystourethrogram (also known as MCUG = micturating cystourethrogram) (can also be fluoroscopy during video-urodynamics study); VUR, vesicoureteral reflux.

with the potential nephrotoxicity and contrast allergy.

Renal/Bladder Sonography

Today, sonography is the preferred method of surveillance imaging of the upper and lower urinary tracts. It has the advantages of no radiation, wide availability, relatively low cost, and little detrimental effect from movement of the child. Sonography is excellent in monitoring renal growth and demonstrating hydronephrosis caused by hostile bladder pressure; its sensitivity for the detection of vesicoureteral reflux (VUR), medical renal disease, renal scarring, and urolithiasis is less than other modalities. Bladder wall thickness has not been found to be a reliable predictor of NLUTD when compared with urodynamic evaluation.[21]

The guidelines mostly agree on the intervals for routine sonography. All recommend imaging soon after birth for congenital NLUTD or after insult in acquired NLUTD to provide a baseline for future comparison. The vast majority starts out with relatively normal upper tracts; a prospective survey of 193 newborns with myelomeningocele found 56% with normal sonograms, 40% with mild hydronephrosis, and only 4% with moderate–severe hydronephrosis.[10] Annual follow-up sonography is the norm among the guidelines with some recommending semiannual in the first 2 years of life and less frequently in school-aged children before

the pubertal growth spurt. The importance of regular imaging is emphasized by a retrospective review of 188 children with myelomeningocele and mean follow-up of 10.4 years demonstrating that 8% of low-risk NLUTD were reclassified to high risk based on new onset hydronephrosis detected on sonography alone.[22] Hydronephrosis has been associated with CKD in a stepwise fashion but has poor sensitivity for mild–moderate reductions in renal function in children with SB.[23]

Cystography

Contrast imaging of the bladder is helpful to better define the severity of NLUTD (**Fig. 1**). As in neuro-normal children, it can detect and grade VUR as well as assess completeness of bladder emptying. Two guidelines recommend bladder imaging by voiding cystourethrography (VCUG) or fluoroscopy during urodynamic evaluation. The same prospective study of newborns with myelomeningocele found 85% to have no VUR, and only 7% of kidneys had dilating (grades 3–5) VUR but does not yet have sufficient follow-up to document changes over time.[10] Hopps and Kropp[22] in their retrospective review found that 9% of low-risk NLUTD developed new VUR over a mean of 10.4 years. In addition, cystography provides useful information regarding bladder shape, trabeculation, diverticula, and bladder outlet competency which can aid in therapeutic decision making.

Dimercaptosuccinic Acid Renal Scintigraphy

[99]Technetium-dimercaptosuccinic acid (DMSA) nuclear renography is the most sensitive test to look for renal scarring and is frequently used in the management of primary VUR. The EAU guidelines recommend its use to obtain a baseline assessment of functioning renal parenchyma in children with NLUTD before any acquired damage by recurrent UTI, secondary VUR, and/or hostile bladder storage pressures. Shiroyanagi and colleagues[24] found that DMSA abnormalities during long-term follow-up correlated only with a history of recurrent febrile UTI and not with other patient or disease parameters. Other guidelines either do not specifically mention it or recommend only if there is significant VUR or suspicion of renal scarring on sonography. The UMPIRE trial, a prospective longitudinal study of newborns with myelomeningocele using a proscribed protocol (but, specifically, not a guideline), uses baseline DMSA scanning in newborns with follow-up scanning at 5 and 9 years of age to assess the success of protocol in preserving renal parenchyma[25] (personal communication with Centers for Disease Control and Prevention, 2023). To date, only one-

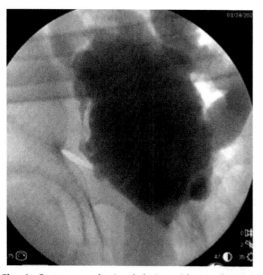

Fig. 1. Cystogram obtained during videourodynamic study of 13-year-old man with a history of surgery for congenital anorectal malformation, urinary incontinence, and recurrent febrile UTI. The bladder is noted to be small in capacity with severe trabeculation. Bilateral VUR is noted with severe dilation on the left.

third of newborns enrolled in the study underwent a baseline DMSA scan due to inconsistent availability of the radiotracer, and an abnormality was noted in just 8%; the study is too young to have sufficient numbers with follow-up imaging.[10]

URODYNAMIC EVALUATION

Urodynamics have been used to correlate neurogenic bladder dysfunction with existing upper tract damage or proactively assess an individual bladder's risk to damage the kidneys in the future.

Historically, detrusor leak point pressure (DLPP) has been the focus as the primary end point based on McGuire's landmark study in 1981 that correlated a DLPP greater than 40 cm H_2O with the findings of VUR or upper tract changes on IVP.[26] Leakage during a voluntary or involuntary contraction does not meet the definition of DLPP, and if no leakage occurs, the end filling pressure serves as a surrogate.[27] Others have used compliance calculated as the ratio of the change in bladder volume divided by the change in bladder pressure

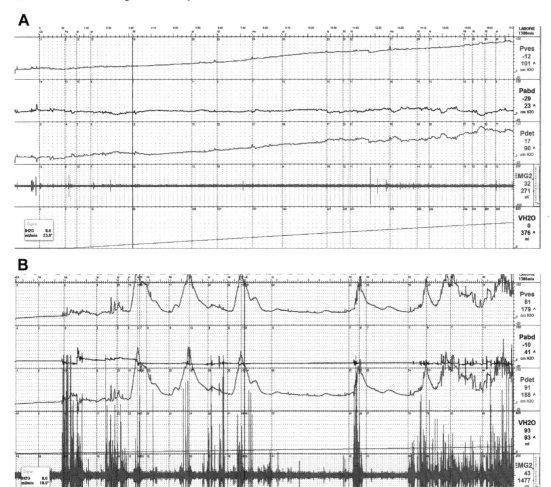

Fig. 2. Urodynamic tracings. (A) *Poor detrusor compliance*: A 13-year-old patient with myelomeningocele has a history of recurrent UTI, bilateral hydronephrosis, and increasing urinary incontinence despite CIC six times daily and combination medical therapy with solifenacin and mirabegron. Tracing shows capacity of 376 mL and detrusor leak point pressure of 56 cm H_2O. At 366 mL, the end filling detrusor pressure was 77 cm H_2O which translates to decreased compliance of 366 mL/77 cm = 4.75. She underwent ileal bladder augmentation and had a resolution of hydronephrosis, incontinence, and UTI. (B) *Neurogenic detrusor overactivity*: A 2-year-old patient with myelomeningocele is on no medications and leaking into his diaper. Filling was stopped at 65 mL due to constant high-volume leakage from repeated uninhibited detrusor contractions of greater than 100 cm H_2O. There was increased pelvic floor EMG activity around the time of contractions, but the start and stop of the EMG activity did not exactly match the detrusor contractions; therefore, he was not felt to have detrusor sphincter dyssynergia. He felt the contractions and moved when they occurred. Owing to the increased magnitude of NDO, he was started on oxybutynin and CIC.

with 10 to 20 mL/cm H_2O as abnormal and less than 10 mL/cm H_2O as severely abnormal to prognosticate potential renal insult.[28] (**Fig. 2**A). Detrusor sphincter dyssynergia (DSD), defined as active contraction, instead of relaxation, of the external urethral sphincter during voiding or uninhibited detrusor contractions, has been thought to be a particularly ominous urodynamic finding. This can be diagnosed by electromyography (EMG) of the sphincter and/or fluoroscopic appearance of the bladder outlet, but the reliability of such measurement is challenging in children.[29] It remains undefined if NDO is predictive of upper tract damage (**Fig. 2**B). VUR complicates urodynamic assessment because it is likely deleterious by transmitting high bladder pressure to the kidneys but also confounding as it can serve as a "pop-off" mechanism to reduce measured detrusor pressures (**Fig. 1**). Real-time fluoroscopy (also known as videourodynamics) can be helpful to identify DSD and VUR as well as show the bladder shape. Trabeculation and/or contracted ("Christmas tree") bladder have been identified as independent predictors of upper tract damage.[30] The prospective UMPIRE study uses urodynamic findings to guide proactive bladder management to better delineate best practices for renal preservation.[25] However, researchers at the 10 centers in this study have found it difficult to reach consensus on urodynamic interpretation driving treatment decisions.[31,32] Clearly, there remains a great deal more work ahead to improve the utility and reliability of urodynamic evaluation of pediatric NLUTD.[33] Future directions may include using artificial intelligence to interpret urodynamic tracings[34] or assessing bladder at home with ambulatory monitoring to provide more realistic assessment of detrusor pressures in the real world, rather than in the artificial testing environment of the urodynamics laboratory.[35,36]

The timing of urodynamic testing is variable.[15] If a neurologic lesion is suspected, as in children with a closed form of SB, nervous system tumor, or persistent incontinence, testing is appropriate before intervention. For those with open form of SB, the child is allowed to fully recover from initial spinal closure before testing is initiated. For those with prenatal closure of SB, testing can be performed when convenient. As a caveat, the prenatal closure has shown little benefit over postnatal closure in terms of reducing the need for future surgical intervention for NLUTD as opposed to its positive effects on ambulation and hydrocephalus, but it has shown higher rates of spontaneous voiding at school age.[37,38] After SCI, NLUTD evolves over time, and it is preferred to wait 3 months after the injury for urodynamic evaluation.

LABORATORY EVALUATION

Serum creatinine is recommended at baseline for newborns with congenital NLUTD by the three guidelines with no consensus from the British Association of Paediatric Urologists statement. Two guidelines recommend routine laboratory follow-up with greater detail in the SBA guidelines. Although intuitive to monitor renal function during development, serum creatinine may be a flawed measure to estimate glomerular filtration rate (GFR) in children with NLUTD. Creatinine is produced by skeletal muscle, and individuals with paraplegia typically have reduced lower extremity muscle mass. Therefore, estimated GFR based on serum creatinine alone may overestimate renal function in this population and be less sensitive to diagnose renal damage and CKD. Serum cystatin C, a renally excreted product of all nucleated cells, seems to be more accurate, and cystatin-based estimated GFR formulas may better reflect true renal function in noncommunity ambulators.[39,40] The UMPIRE trial aims to compare estimated GFR with actual direct determination of GFR in children with NLUTD secondary to SB, but few of the cohort has reached the age for GFR testing[25] (personal communication with Centers for Disease Control and Prevention, 2023).

Testing urine for UTI in individuals with NLUTD is similarly problematic. CIC is the norm for many with NLUTD—used in over 76% of adolescents and adults with myelomeningocele,[6] and most will have bacteriuria. Therefore, the presence of bacteria in the urine does not equate to UTI but may simply reflect urinary tract colonization.[41] The SBA guidelines provide specific definitions to diagnose UTI: a specimen should be obtained by sterile catheterization and have a positive urinalysis (> trace nitrite or leukocyte esterase on dipstick, > 5 or > 10 white blood cell per high-powered field microscopy on centrifuged or uncentrifuged specimens, respectively) and positive urine culture (>50,000 or >100,000 colony forming units/mL on catheterized or clean voided specimen, respectively).[12,13]

CLEAN INTERMITTENT CATHETERIZATION

In 1972, Lapides and colleagues published the revolutionary study that first described CIC in the management of NLUTD. CIC decreases upper tract injury and UTI by allowing safe regular emptying of bladders unable to empty spontaneously, thus reducing urinary tract distention that can increase bladder wall pressure and ischemia if bladder pressures exceed diastolic blood pressure.[17,42]

Controversy exists around the age at which CIC should be started depending if one is using proactive or expectant management.[19,43] The EAU guidelines take the most proactive approach, advocating for early initiation of CIC (in the neonatal period in congenital cases) to ensure regular bladder emptying.[14] This assumes that all bladders are hostile until proven otherwise, but they do add the caveat that initiation can be delayed if the outlet/sphincter is underactive or weak because urine will leak out before bladder storage pressures reach deleterious levels. The SBA and ICCS guidelines take an approach dictated more by urodynamic or imaging findings worrisome for hostile bladder, although the latter do suggest initiation as soon as feasible after SCI or until urodynamics can be performed in congenital cases if bladder emptying is suboptimal.[12,13]

Proponents argue that proactive management provides better family and patient acceptance of CIC, improved long-term renal outcomes, and decreased need for future surgical reconstruction.[44–46] The use of CIC and medication is dictated by early performance of urodynamic studies and imaging and can be stopped if bladder residuals are low or the bladder is deemed safe.

On the contrary, proponents of expectant management recommend initiating CIC only when there is evidence of upper tract changes, recurrent UTI, or bothersome incontinence. CIC, therefore, is not universally initiated in the neonatal period and only started when imaging studies show upper tract changes.[19,43] Proponents argue that upper tract changes, when caught early, are reversible. Moreover, this approach avoids unnecessary familial stress caused by CIC and morbidity of treatment.[46,47] Interestingly, studies have shown higher rates of vesicostomy in patients on expectant management, as well higher bladder augmentation rates.[20,44–46]

Because of the importance of gaining independence, the SBA guidelines recommend that caregivers start involving the child in the process of CIC as early as 3 to 5 years of age.[12,13]

PHARMACOTHERAPY

Along with CIC, pharmacotherapy is an integral part of management of NLUTD. The mode of pharmacotherapy should be determined by (1) predominant type of NLUTD (*storage dysfunction*: NDO, high bladder storage pressure, and weak outlet vs *voiding dysfunction*: detrusor underactivity, increased outlet resistance, and DSD), (2) type of formulation (oral liquid or pill, intravesical, or transdermal), and (3) tolerance of side effects. Owing to the many innovations in pharmacotherapy for NLUTD over several decades, clinicians must stay abreast of the growing options (**Table 2**).

The first-line pharmacologic management for NLUTD is anticholinergic agents that block muscarinic receptors with some being highly selective for the M2/M3 receptors in the bladder.[15,48] Along with CIC, proactive proponents start anticholinergic medication early in infancy to further reduce bladder pressure, improve detrusor compliance, and decrease morbidity.[19,45] The EAU guidelines are most proactive in recommending pharmacotherapy if NDO is suspected. The ICCS recommends anticholinergic medications if high-grade VUR, high filling pressures, or NDO are noted on initial evaluation, along with CIC.[14,16] The SBA guidelines also recommend medication if hostile bladder characteristics are noted on urodynamics but, otherwise, are more expectant only if recurrent UTI, upper tract changes, or mixed incontinence occur.[12,13] Studies have shown that these agents improve urodynamic parameters, including increasing bladder capacity and decreasing storage pressures in infants, and may lead to bladder wall remodeling.[48,49] Side effects of anticholinergic medications include dry mouth, facial flushing, dry eyes, and constipation, such that many young patients cannot tolerate them.[50]

Oxybutynin is the most commonly prescribed anticholinergic medication in part because it was the only antimuscarinic that was Food and Drug Administration (FDA)-approved in pediatric patients until recently. Oxybutynin is a tertiary amine antimuscarinic with affinity to M3 receptors. Oral dosing for the liquid form is 0.2 mg/kg TID-QID. Extended release pills have been shown to have better side effect profile than immediate release tablets.[51] The transdermal route (patch or gel) has been shown to be well-tolerated and an effective alternative to oral oxybutynin.[50] Intravesical administration of oxybutynin is another route with decreased side effects as it, similar to the transdermal preparation, bypasses hepatic metabolism. Studies have shown promising results with intravesical administration with increased maximum bladder capacity and decreased pressures; however, it can be challenging to give as pills must be crushed and instilled into the bladder via catheter.[52]

Tolterodine is another tertiary amine antimuscarinic which has been shown to be effective and well-tolerated among pediatric patients. It only minimally crosses the blood–brain barrier and has a favorable side effect profile. The immediate release (BID) formulated only comes in a pill form which must be crushed, but the extended release form comes in a capsule that can be opened.[53] Fesoterodine is another tertiary amine

Table 2
Pharmacotherapy options for neurogenic lower urinary tract dysfunction

Medication	Dose	Side Effects
Antimuscarinics		
Oxybutynin[a] (3° amine)	IR 5 mg tablets q6–8h Liquid 5 mg/5 mL	Dry mouth, dry eyes, constipation, blurry vision, urinary retention, confusion
	ER 5 mg, 10 mg, 15 mg Patch (Oxytrol) 3.7 mg	ER has less side effects Localized skin reaction may have less systemic effects
	Gel (Gelnique)	Same
Tolterodine (3° amine)	IR 2–4 mg BID (Can be crushed) ER 2–8 mg daily Capsule (can be opened)	Same as oxybutynin ER has less side effects
Fesoterodine[a] (3° amine)	4–8 mg daily	May have less side effects than tolterodine
Solifenacin (3° amine)	5–10 mg tablets daily Liquid 5 mg/5 ml	Same as oxybutynin
Darifenacin (3° amine)	7.5–15 mg tablets	Same as solifenacin
Trospium (4° amine)	IR 20 mg BID	Does not cross blood–brain barrier, CNS side effects may be less
	ER 20–60 mg daily	Less than IR tablets
B3 selective receptor agonist		
Mirabegron[a]	25–50 mg daily	Hypertension, dyspepsia
Vibegron	75 mg daily	
Tricyclic antidepressants		
Imipramine[b]	10–45 mg divided BID/TID	Dizziness, drowsiness, dry mouth, constipation, blurred vision, nightmares, dyspepsia, lethal cardiac arrhythmia at high doses

Abbreviations: ER, extended release; IR, immediate release.
[a] FDA-approved for use in children (not all approved for all ages).
[b] Has adrenergic characteristics.

antimuscarinic with the same active metabolite as tolterodine and may have fewer side effects than tolterodine. It has been shown to be safe and tolerable in children.[54] Solifenacin is an additional tertiary amine antimuscarinic with affinity for the M3 receptor and has been shown to improved bladder capacity, reduce overactivity, and improve continence. It seems safe for pediatric patients and also comes in a liquid form which can be quite expensive.[55] Trospium, a quaternary amine antimuscarinic, does not cross the blood–brain barrier and has minimal affinity for M1 receptors, so side effect profile is low.[56]

Beta-3-agonists that stimulate adrenergic receptors to relax the detrusor muscle offer an alternative to anticholinergic medical therapy for NLUTID with fewer side effects. Mirabegron, now FDA-approved in children with NDO, comes in a pill and liquid suspension so is a good option for the young patient. Early prospective data show promising results with mirabegron in NLUTD management.[57,58] There is a hypothetical risk of hypertension with mirabegron use, but pediatric data are not well validated. Vibegron is currently being investigated for pediatric NLUTD.

Tricyclic antidepressants (TCAs), such as imipramine, were historically used in NLUTD but today have a limited scope in pediatric population given their low therapeutic–toxicity index. TCA have been shown to relax the detrusor muscle by acting as muscarinic receptor antagonist and have weak adrenergic effects to tighten the bladder neck that may improve continence. Overdose of TCAs can result in cardiac arrhythmia.[59]

Alpha-adrenergic blockers, such terazosin or tamsulosin, can be used for NLUTD with high outlet resistance at the bladder neck. These medications help to relax the smooth muscle in the internal sphincteric complex (but not the external skeletal muscle sphincter) to improve voiding in those patients with volitional control who do not have issues with urine storage but have poor emptying. Side effects include hypotension, dizziness, and headache. Tamsulosin is more selective and has higher affinity to alpha-adrenergic receptors in the urinary tract.[60,61]

BOTULINUM TOXIN

Intravesical botulinum toxin (BTA) is a next line option for treatment of NDO and decreased bladder compliance in NLUTD patients who cannot achieve continence or safe storage pressures with oral pharmacotherapy. BTA is a neurotoxin protein produced by the bacteria *Clostridium botulinum*; it acts by inhibiting acetylcholine release resulting in flaccid muscle paralysis. The first reported use of BTA in children with NLUTD in 2002 proved to be safe and effective,[62] and it has become increasingly popular. Interestingly, it was only as recent as 2021 that FDA-approved BTA for use in pediatric NDO.[63] Typically, 100 to 200 IU are injected in 10 to 30 intradetrusor sites (refer to package insert). In pediatric patients, the procedure typically requires general anesthesia as most do not tolerate an awake cystoscopy; however, the repeated need for anesthesia can be prohibitive.

BTA has been proven to be efficacious as the next-line treatment for NDO and is mentioned in the EAU guidelines. Systematic reviews show improvement in urinary incontinence episodes by 32-100%, increase in bladder capacity of 27-162%, and increased compliance of 28-176%.[64,65] Injection of BTA may allow approximately 25% of patients to discontinue antimuscarinic therapy after the first injection.[66] Duration of response varied from 6 to 10.5 months; thus, parents and patients must be made aware that they will likely require repeat procedures.[65,67] Nonetheless, BTA has shown promising results with minimal side effects and is a good option for patients who experience intolerable side effects of pharmacotherapy or do not achieve satisfactory results. This may allow them to either avoid surgical reconstruction altogether or, at least, delay it. The adverse effects of BTA include hematuria, UTI, and urinary retention, the latter of which is not problematic in those on CIC.[67]

NEUROSTIMULATION

Neuromodulation is another option for some children with NLUTD. The data are limited as most studies have small sample size, and the indications are narrow. The Interstim sacral neuromodulation device involves permanent electrical stimulation of the sacral nerves at S3 level using an implantable device that "shocks" nerves to modulate bladder function. Sacral neuromodulation was initially used for non-NLUTD bladder patients with urinary retention or detrusor overactivity. A small study in children with NLUTD showed modest improvement of bladder capacity and decrease in DLPP with neuromodulation, but 7% needed revision of the device.[68] The role of sacral neuromodulation in NLUTD is limited, as lead placement in individuals with prior spinal cord surgery can pose challenging.

There have been studies looking at transurethral intravesical bladder electrostimulation with promising increases in bladder capacity noted.[69] However, this technique is labor-intensive and has not garnered wide acceptance over the decades.

RECONSTRUCTIVE SURGERY

Primary indications for reconstructive surgery for NLUTD are the presence of renal deterioration despite maximal medical management, desire to achieve social continence, and desire to achieve independence as children transition to adults. The EAU guidelines, being more comprehensive than the others, address surgical management of NLUTD.[14] Before the introduction of CIC, incontinent urinary diversion was the gold standard in patients with hostile, low compliance bladders.[8] These include vesicostomy, ileal conduit, ileovesicostomy, or incontinent reservoirs. Although these procedures were mostly successful in preserving renal function, they were often detrimental to QOL as these children grew up with an external urostomy bag. With the advent of CIC, continent surgical reconstruction with or without the use of catheterizable channels has gained widespread popularity and has provided improved QOL in these patients.

Vesicostomy

Vesicostomy is still a preferred option in young children with hostile NLUTD in whom CIC is not feasible for anatomic or social reasons or cannot be sufficiently managed with pharmacotherapy. With expectant management, higher rates of vesicostomy have been reported as the introduction of CIC at a later age in life can be challenging for both patients and parents.[20,22] Vesicostomy can be reversed and often buys time until the child is mature enough or family is ready for undergo surgical reconstruction necessitating CIC. The complications of vesicostomy include stenosis and bladder prolapse requiring revision. Daily catheterization of the stoma may prevent stenosis and "introduces" CIC to the child and caregivers.

Bladder Augmentation

Enterocystoplasty (bladder augmentation with intestinal segment) is the first-line surgical management for bladders with low capacity and/or poor compliance that have failed medical management.[14] A patch of detubularized intestine, typically ileum or sigmoid colon, is added to bladder to increase its size, creating a large, low-pressure reservoir for urine storage that must be emptied via CIC.[1] If patient has an incompetent bladder outlet, then a bladder neck reconstruction (BNR) with or without a sling should be performed for provide urinary continence, if so desired.[14] If BNR is performed, CIC via urethra is usually no longer possible, and a continent catheterizable channel using the appendix (Mitrofanoff) or retubularized segment of ileum (Monti) can be created.[1,14]

Enterocystoplasty is highly effective but not without significant short-term and long-term complications.[1] These are long procedures with high morbidity. Short-term complications include infection, bowel leak, urine leak, and postoperative ileus. Long-term complications include bladder stone formation, excess mucous production, recurrent UTI, bowel obstruction, electrolyte imbalance, osteopenia, and bladder perforation.[1] Bladder perforation is a potentially fatal complication that requires emergent surgical attention. Vitamin B_{12} deficiency can result if terminal ileum is used, and hyperchloremic hypokalemic metabolic acidosis can occur with both ileal and colonic augmentation. SBA and EAU guidelines suggest lifelong laboratory screening for electrolyte and B_{12} alternations.[12–14,70] Late malignant development has been noted after enterocystoplasty, so guidelines address the need for regular screening cystoscopy beginning as early as 10 years postoperatively, but some question the utility of this practice.[71] Stomal stenosis, stricture, and inability to catheterize are common complications of continent catheterizable channels. In particular, Monti channels, irregularly constructed by their nature, can be more challenging to catheterize over time as they can become dilated and redundant from the force of catheterization.

Because augmentation with intestine carries a significant risk for complications, some have advocated autoaugmentation or detrusorectomy (with or without demucosalized enteric segment coverage) to achieve the same benefit.[72] These procedures are rarely used as long-term outcomes have been proven to be inferior to enterocystoplasty with increased rates of incontinence and poor compliance.[73]

Some have proposed the ureteral augmentation for nonenteric bladder enlargement. This is only possible in very specialized situations in which there is a nonfunctioning kidney with ureteral dilation. The ureteral dilation must be significant enough to provide an adequate patch to the bladder. One study showed a 76% long-term success rate.[74]

Bladder Neck Procedures

Incompetent bladder outlet due to intrinsic sphincter deficiency is a common feature of NLUTD. Although this creates a low-pressure urinary system, it can be devastating for patients who desire social continence. Injectable bulking agents are least invasive option to increase outlet resistance. There are several compounds available, but the most commonly used is dextranomer/hyaluronic acid (Deflux) (off-label indication). Efficacy in retrograde injection is limited with decreased efficacy over time. Antegrade injection via a continent catheterizable channel, if present, has been shown to be superior to the retrograde approach.[75,76]

BNR techniques predominantly work by elongating and narrowing the urethral lumen to increase outlet resistance. Alternatively, or in combination with BNR, bladder neck slings can be placed to increase outlet resistance of the urethra, but regardless of techniques used, success rates of bladder neck procedures rarely exceed 70%.[1,77] Slings can be made of autologous fascia (commonly, rectus sheath), biological graft, or synthetic material, and various sling configurations exist. Bladder neck sling (in combination with continent catheterizable channel) has been reported without augmentation in bladders with sphincter deficiency but adequate capacity and compliance.[78] However, longer term follow-up of this practice has shown that the bladder may decompensate after outlet resistance is increased, and up to 30% require later augmentation; therefore, these patients require careful selection and follow-up.[77]

Artificial urinary sphincter (AUS) is another option to increase outlet resistance while still maintaining the ability to perform CIC per urethra in select patients. In younger males and all females, the AUS cuff should be placed around the bladder neck, whereas in older males, less invasive placement around bulbar urethra is possible. Continence rates range from 63% to 86%, but the need for revision ranges from 16% to 61 with erosion of the cuff noted in 16% to 20%.[79–81]

BOWEL MANAGEMENT AND SEXUALITY

Although beyond the scope of this article on NLUTD management, the guidelines reinforce that bowel management cannot be ignored in those with neurogenic bowel dysfunction, as fecal incontinence can be more detrimental to QOL than urinary incontinence.[82] Sexual dysfunction is common in this population and should be evaluated and addressed as patients progress through adolescence and into adulthood.[83,84]

CLINICS CARE POINTS

- Most guidelines favor proactive management of NLUTD.
- Routine imaging by US and laboratory monitoring of renal function is required for proactive or reactive management.
- Urodynamic evaluaton of NLUTD is a critical tool in management of NLUTD but may be used proactively or reactively.
- Pharmacotherapy, CIC, and/or surgical intervention are used in a step-wise approach for management of hostile bladders, poor bladder emptying, and/or urinary incontinence.

DISCLOSURE

Dr J.S. Wiener is a funded researcher by the Centers for Disease Control and Prevention, United States for the National Spina Bifida Patient Registry and the UMPIRE protocol. He is presently conducting research for Urovant Sciences, Ltd. Dr R. Chaudhry has no conflicts to report.

REFERENCES

1. Thomas JC, Clayton DB, Adams MC. Lower Urinary Tract Reconstruction. In: Partin AW, Dmochoski RR, Kavoussi LR, et al, editors. Campbell-walsh-wein urology. 12th edition. Philadelphia: Elsevier; 2021. p. 680–713.
2. Shin M, Besser LM, Siffel C, et al. Prevalence of spina bifida among children and adolescents in 10 regions in the United States. Pediatrics 2010;126: 274–9.
3. Mai CT, Isenburg JL, Canfield M, et al. National population-based estimates for major birth defects, 2010-2014. Birth Defects Res 2019;111:1420–35.
4. Mathews TJ, Honein MA, Erickson JD. Spina bifida and anencephaly prevalence – United States, 1991-2001. MMWR Recomm Rep 2002;51:9–11.
5. What is spina bifida? In: National Center on Birth Defects and Developmental Disabilities. Centers for Disease Control and Prevention Available at: https://www.cdc.gov/ncbddd/spinabifida/facts. Accessed February 6, 2023.
6. Wiener JS, Suson KD, Castillo J, et al. Bladder management and continence in adults with spina bifida: results from the National Spina Bifida Patient Registry 2009-2015. J Urol 2018;200:187–93.
7. Nalbandyan M, Howley MM, Cunniff CM, et al. Descriptive and risk factor analysis of nonsyndromic sacral agenesis: National Birth Defects Prevention Study, 1997-2011. Am J Med Genet 2019;179:1799–814.
8. Smith ED. Urinary prognosis in spina bifida. J Urol 1972;108:815–7.
9. Strine AC, Misseri R, Szymanski KM, et al. Assessing health related benefit after reconstruction for urinary and fecal incontinence in children: a parental perspective. J Urol 2015;193:2073–8.
10. Tanaka ST, Paramsothy P, Thibadeau J, et al. Baseline urinary tract imaging in infants enrolled in the UMPIRE protocol for children with spina bifida. J Urol 2019;201:1193–8.
11. Struwe S, Thibadeau J, Kelly MS, et al. Establishing the first community-centered spina bifida research agenda. J Pediatr Urol 2022;18:800e1–7.
12. Joseph DB, Baille S, Baum MA, et al. Urology. In: Guidelines for the Care of People Living with Spina Bifida. Spina Bifida Association. 2018, pp. 162-175. Available at: https://www.spinabifidaassociation.org/guidelines/. Accessed February 4, 2023.
13. Joseph DB, Baum MA, Tanaka ST, et al. Urologic guidelines for the care and management of people with spina bifida. J Pediatr Rehabil Med 2020;13: 479–89.
14. Radmayr C, Bogaert G, Burgu B et al. EAU Guidelines on Pediatric Urology. 2022. Pp. 49- 63. Available at: https://uroweb.org/guidelines/paediatric-urology/chapter/the-guideline. Accessed February 4, 2023.
15. Lee B, Featherstone N, Nagappan G, et al. British Association of Paediatric Urologists consensus statement on management of neuropathic bladder. J Pediatr Urol 2016;12:76–87.
16. Bauer SB, Austin PF, Rawashdeh YF, et al. International Children's Continence Society's Recommendations for Initial Diagnostic Evaluation and Follow-up in Congenital Neuropathic Bladder and Bowel Dysfunction in Children. Neurourol Urodyn 2012;31:610–4.
17. Lapides J, Diokno AC, Silber JC, et al. Clean, intermittent self-catheterizaton in the treatment of urinary tract disease. J Urol 1972;107:458–61.
18. Diokno AC, Lapides J. Oxybutynin: a new drug with analgesic and anticholinergic properties. J Urol 1972;108:307–9.
19. Hobbs KT, Krischak M, Tejwani R, et al. The importance of early diagnosis and management of pediatric neurogenic bladder dysfunction. Res Report Urol 2021;13:647–57.
20. Teichman JM, Scherz HC, Kim KD, et al. An alternative approach to myelodysplasia management: aggressive observation and prompt intervention. J Urol 1994;152:807–11.

21. Kim WJ, Shiroyanagi Y, Yamazaki Y. Can bladder wall thickness predict videourodynamic findings in children with spina bifida? J Urol 2015;194: 180–3.

22. Hopps CV, Kropp KA. Preservation of renal function in children with myelomeningocele managed with basic newborn evaluation and close follow up. J Urol 2003;169:305–8.

23. Chu DI, Balmert LC, Chen L, et al. Diagnostic test characteristics of ultrasound based hydronephrosis in identifying low kidney function in young patients with spina bifida: a retrospective cohort study. J Urol 2021;205:1180–8.

24. Shiroyanagi Y, Suzuki M, Matsuno D, et al. The significance of ^{99}mtechnetium dimercaptosuccinic acid renal scan in children with spina bifida during long-term followup. J Urol 2009;181:2262–6.

25. Routh JC, Cheng EY, Austin JC, et al. Design and methodologic considerations of the Centers for Disease Control and Prevention Urologic and Renal Protocol for the newborn and young child with spina bifida. J Urol 2016;196:1728–34.

26. McGuire EJ, Woodside JR, Borden TA, et al. Prognostic value of urodynamic testing in myelodysplastic patients. J Urol 1981;125:205–9.

27. Austin PF, Bauer SB, Bower W, et al. The standardization of terminology of lower urinary tract function in children and adolescents: report update from the standardization committee of the International Children's Continence Society. Neurol Urodyn 2016;35: 471–8.

28. Galloway NTM, Mekras JA, Helms M, et al. An objective score to predict upper tract deterioration in myelodysplasia. J Urol 1991;145:535–7.

29. Dudley AG, Adams MC, Brock JW, et al. Interrater reliability in interpretation of neuropathic pediatric urodynamic tracings: an expanded multicenter study. J Urol 2018;199:1337–43.

30. Timberlake MD, Jacobs MA, Kern AJ, et al. Streamlining risk stratification in infants and young children with spina dysraphism: vesicoureteral reflux and/or bladder trabeculations outperforms other urodynamic findings for predicting adverse outcomes. J Pediatr Urol 2018;14:319e1–7.

31. Yerkes EB, Cheng E, Wiener JS, et al. Translating pediatric urodynamics from clinic into collaborative research: lessons and recommendations from the UMPIRE study group. J Pediatr Urol 2021;17:716–25.

32. Tanaka ST, Yerkes EB, Routh JC, et al. Urodynamic characteristics of neurogenic bladder in newborns with myelomeningocele and refinement of the definition of bladder hostility: Findings from the UMPIRE multi-center study. J Pediatr Urol 2021;17: 726–32.

33. Weaver JK, Weiss DA, Aghababian A, et al. Why are pediatric urologists unable to predict renal deterioration using urodynamics? A focused narrative review of the shortcomings of the literature. J Pediatr Urol 2022;18:493–8.

34. Hobbs KT, Choe N, Aksenov LI, et al. Machine learning for urodynamic detection of detrusor overactivity. Urology 2022;159:247–54.

35. Cooper CS, Bonnett MA, Ortman CE, et al. Pilot study of a home use cystomanometer in patients with a neurogenic bladder. J Pediatr Urol 2022;18: 466–8.

36. Huen KH, Chamberlin JD, Macaraeg A, et al. Home bladder pressure measurements correlate with urodynamic storage pressures and high-grade hydronephrosis in children with spina bifida. J Pediat Urol 2022;18:503e1–7.

37. Adzick NS, Thom EA, Spong CY, et al. A randomized trial of prenatal versus postnatal repair of myelomeningocele. N Engl J Med 2011;364:993–1004.

38. Brock JW, Thomas JC, Baskin LA, et al. Effect of prenatal repair of myelomeningocele on urologic outcomes at school age. J Urol 2019;202:812–8.

39. Chu DI, Balmert LC, Arkin CM, et al. Estimated kidney in children and young adults with spina bifida: a retrospective cohort study. Neurol Urodyn 2019;38: 1907–14.

40. Werneburg GT, Hettel D, Jeong S, et al. Estimated glomerular filtration rate using cystatin C is a more sensitive marker for kidney dysfunction in nonweighbearing individuals. J Urol 2023;209:391–8.

41. Madden-Fuentes RJ, McNamara ER, Lloyd JC, et al. Variation in definitions of urinary tract infections in spina bifida patients: a systematic review. Pediatrics 2013;132:132–9.

42. Mehrotra RML. An experimental study of the vesical circulation during distention and in cystitis. J Path Bact 1953;66:79.

43. Snow-Lisy DC, Yerkes EB, Cheng EY. Update on Urological Management of Spina Bifida from Prenatal Diagnosis to Adulthood. J Urol 2015;(2):194–288.

44. Edelstein RA, Bauer SB. The long term response of neonates with myelodysplasia treated proactively with intermittent catheterization and anticholinergic therapy. J Urol 1995;154:1500.

45. Wu HY, Baskin LS, Kogan BA. Neurogenic bladder dysfunction due to myelomeningocele: neonatal versus childhood treatment. J Urol 1997;157(6): 2295–7.

46. Kaufman AM, Ritchey ML, Roberts AC, et al. Decreased bladder compliance in patients with myelomeningocele treated with radiological observation. J Urol 1996;156:2031.

47. Klose AG, Sackett CK, Mesrobian HG. Management of children with myelodysplasia: urological alternatives. J Urol 1990;144(6):1446.

48. Lee AS, Viseshsindh W, Long CJ, et al. How early is early? Effect of oxybutynin on bladder dynamics within the first year of life in patients with spina bifida. J Pediatr Urol 2020;16(2):168.e1-6.

49. Liu Q, Luo D, Yang T, et al. Protective effects of anti-muscarinics on the bladder remodeling after bladder outlet obstruction. Cell Physiol Biochem 2017;44(3):907–19.

50. Cartwright PC, Coplen DE, Kogan BA, et al. Efficacy and safety of transdermal and oral oxybutynin in children with neurogenic detrusor overactivity. J Urol 2009;182(4):1548–54.

51. Katrin Y, Kogan BA. Preliminary study of the safety and efficacy of extended-release oxybutynin in children. Urology 2002;59(3):428–32.

52. Guerra LA, Moher D, Sampson M, et al. Intravesical oxybutynin for children with poorly compliant neurogenic bladder: a systematic review. J Urol 2008; 180(3):1091–7.

53. Reddy PP, Borgstein NG, Nijman RJ, et al. Long-term efficacy and safety of tolterodine in children with neurogenic detrusor overactivity. J Pediatr Urol 2008;4(6):428–33.

54. Malhotra B, El-Tahtawy A, Wang EQ, et al. Dose-escalating study of the pharmacokinetics and tolerability of fesoterodine in children with overactive bladder. J Pediatr Urol 2012;8(4):336–42.

55. Bolduc S, Moore K, Nadeau G, et al. Prospective open label study of solifenacin for overactive bladder in children. J Urol 2010;184(4 Suppl): 1668–73.

56. Lopez Pereira P, Miguelez C, Caffarati J, et al. Trospium chloride for the treatment of detrusor instability in children. J Urol 2003;170(5):1978–81.

57. Blais AS, Nadeau G, Moore K, et al. Prospective pilot study of mirabegron in pediatric patients with overactive bladder. Eur Urol 2016;70(1):9–13.

58. Park JS, Lee YS, Lee CN, et al. Efficacy and safety of mirabegron, a β3-adrenoceptor agonist, for treating neurogenic bladder in pediatric patients with spina bifida: a retrospective pilot study. World J Urol 2019;37:1665–70.

59. Cameron AP, Clemens JQ, Latini JM, et al. Combination drug therapy improves compliance of the neurogenic bladder. J Urol 2009;182(3):1062–7.

60. Husmann, Douglas A. Use of sympathetic alpha antagonists in the management of pediatric urologic disorders. Curr Opin Urol 2006;16(4):277–82.

61. Kroll P, Gajewska E, Zachwieja JE, et al. An Evaluation of the Efficacy of Selective Alpha-Blockers in the Treatment of Children with Neurogenic Bladder Dysfunction—Preliminary Findings. J Env Res Pub Health 2016;13(3):321.

62. Schulte-Baukloh H, Knispel HH, Stolze T, et al. Repeated botulinum-A toxin injections in treatment of children with neurogenic detrusor overactivity. Urology 2005;66(4):865–70.

63. Botox® (onabotulinumtoxinA) receives FDA approval for pediatric detrusor overactivity associated with a neurologic condition. [press release]. North Chicago, IL: AbbVie; 2021.

64. Hascoet J, Manunta A, Brochard C, et al. Outcomes of intra-detrusor injections of botulinum toxin in patients with spina bifida: a systematic review. Neurourol Urodyn 2017;36(3):557–64.

65. Naqvi S, Clothier J, Wright A, et al. Urodynamic outcomes in children after single and multiple injections for overactive and low compliance neurogenic bladder treated with abobotulinum toxin A. J Urol 2020;203(2):413–9.

66. Figueroa V, Romao R, Pippi Salle JL, et al. Single-center experience with botulinum toxin endoscopic detrusor injection for the treatment of congenital neuropathic bladder in children: effect of dose adjustment, multiple injections, and avoidance of reconstructive procedures. J Pediatr Urol 2014; 10(2):368–73.

67. Hascoet J, Peyronnet B, Forin V, et al. Intradetrusor injections of botulinum toxin type A in children with spina bifida: a multicenter study. Urology 2018; 116:161–7.

68. Guys JM, Haddad M, Planche D, et al. Sacral neuromodulation for neurogenic bladder dysfunction in children. J Urol 2004;172(4):1673–6.

69. Kaplan WE, Richards TW, Richards I. Intravesical transurethral bladder stimulation to increase bladder capacity. J Urol 1989;142(2):600–2.

70. Gilbert SM, Hensle TW. Metabolic consequences and long-term complications of enterocystoplasty in children: a review. J Urol 2005;173(4):1080–6.

71. Higuchi TT, Fox JA, Husmann DA. Annual endoscopy and urine cytology for the surveillance of bladder tumors after enterocystoplasty for congenital bladder anomalies. J Urol 2011;186(5):1791–5.

72. Cartwright PC, Snow BW. Bladder autoaugmentation: partial detrusor excision to augment the bladder without use of bowel. J Urol 1989;142(4): 1050–3.

73. MacNeily AE, Afshar K, Coleman GU, et al. Autoaugmentation by detrusor myotomy: its lack of effectiveness in the management of congenital neuropathic bladder. J Urol 2003;170(4):1643–6.

74. Johal NS, Hamid R, Aslam Z, et al. Ureterocystoplasty: long-term functional results. J Urol 2008; 179(6):2373–6.

75. Alova I, Margaryan M, Bernuy M, et al. Long-term effects of endoscopic injection of dextranomer/hyaluronic acid based implants for treatment of urinary incontinence in children with neurogenic bladder. J Urol 2012;188(5):1905–9.

76. Dean GE, Kirsch AJ, Packer MG, et al. Antegrade and retrograde endoscopic dextranomer/hyaluronic Acid bladder neck bulking for pediatric incontinence. J Urol 2007;178(2):652–5.

77. Grimsby GM, Menon V, Schlomer BJ, et al. Long-term outcomes of bladder neck reconstruction without augmentation cystoplasty in children. J Urol 2016;195(1):155–61.

78. Snodgrass WT, Elmore J, Adams R. Bladder neck sling and appendicovesicostomy without augmentation for neurogenic incontinence in children. J Urol 2007;177(4):1510–4.

79. Catti M, Lortat-Jacob S, Morineau M, et al. Artificial urinary sphincter in children—voiding or emptying? An evaluation of functional results in 44 patients. J Urol 2008;180(2):690–3.

80. Herndon CD, Rink RC, Shaw MB, et al. The Indiana experience with the artificial urinary sphincter in children and young adults. J Urol 2003;169(2):650–4.

81. Simeoni J, Guys JM, Mollard P, et al. Artificial urinary sphincter implantation for neurogenic bladder: a multi-institutional study in 107 children. Br J Urol 1996;78(2):287–93.

82. Szymanski KM, Cain MP, Whittam B, et al. All incontinence is not created equal: impact of urinary and fecal incontinence on quality of life in adults with spina bifida. J Urol 2017;197(3):885–91.

83. Steur CS, Corona L, Smith JE, et al. Sexual function of men and women with spina bifida: a scoping literature review. Sex Med Rev 2021;9:244–66.

84. Hughes TL, Simmons KL, Tejwani R, et al. Sexual function and dysfunction in individuals with spina bifida: a systematic review. Urology 2021;156:308–19.

Differences of Sex Development
Current Issues and Controversies

Emilie K. Johnson, MD, MPH[a,b,*], Jax Whitehead, MD[c,d],
Earl Y. Cheng, MD[a,b]

KEYWORDS

- Disorders of sex development • Intersex persons • Diagnosis • Patient care team
- Patient advocacy

KEY POINTS

- Differences of sex development (DSD) represent a broad range of conditions that are cared for by a multidisciplinary team that includes surgical specialists, endocrinologists, behavioral health professionals, and genetics experts.
- DSD nomenclature is controversial, as is whether certain conditions (particularly proximal hypospadias and congenital adrenal hyperplasia) should be classified as DSDs.
- Diagnostic evaluation of suspected DSD includes physical exam, ultrasound imaging, and endocrine testing, with an increased emphasis on genetic testing as options expand.
- For patients with DSD who are at increased risk for gonadal tumors, management options are individualized based on diagnosis, age, expected hormonal and fertility potential, and patient/family goals.
- External genital surgical techniques have advanced significantly over the last several decades; the timing of these procedures is currently the most controversial aspect of DSD care, with widely different perspectives presented by patients, families, and medical professionals.

INTRODUCTION

Differences of sex development (DSD, also referred to as intersex conditions) are conditions in which the development of chromosomal, gonadal, or anatomic sex is not typically male or female.[1] A few of the most common examples include congenital adrenal hyperplasia (CAH), various forms of gonadal dysgenesis, partial and complete androgen insensitivity syndromes (PAIS and CAIS), and ovotesticular DSD. The approach to DSD care has changed substantially over the last two decades. The goal of this review is to provide an update on current issues and controversies related to the care of individuals with DSD.

Nomenclature

The terminology used to describe DSD has evolved over time, and there is still no standard set of terms that has been agreed upon by clinicians, patients, and advocates. The term "disorder

[a] Division of Urology, Ann & Robert H. Lurie Children's Hospital of Chicago, 225 East Chicago Avenue, Box 24, Chicago, IL 60611, USA; [b] Department of Urology, Northwestern University Feinberg School of Medicine, 676 North Saint Clair, Suite 2300, Chicago, IL, 60611, USA; [c] Division of Endocrinology, Ann & Robert H. Lurie Children's Hospital of Chicago, 225 East Chicago Avenue, Box 54, Chicago, IL 60611, USA; [d] Department of Pediatrics, Northwestern University Feinberg School of Medicine, 225 East Chicago Avenue, Box 86, Chicago, IL 60611, USA
* Corresponding author. Division of Urology, Ann & Robert H. Lurie Children's Hospital of Chicago, 225 East Chicago Avenue, Box 24, Chicago, IL 60611-2605.
E-mail address: ekjohnson@luriechildrens.org

Urol Clin N Am 50 (2023) 433–446
https://doi.org/10.1016/j.ucl.2023.04.010
0094-0143/23/© 2023 Elsevier Inc. All rights reserved.

of sex development" was part of a set of new nomenclature developed by a multidisciplinary group of stakeholders and was published through the 2006 "Chicago Consensus Statement".[1] The goal was to provide diagnostically accurate terms that reflected updated molecular genetics knowledge and lent clarity related to research and communication.[1] **Table 1** contrasts previous and revised nomenclature. This most updated medical nomenclature (**Table 2**) separates DSD diagnoses first by chromosomes, and then by whether the diagnosis is related to gonadal development or androgen synthesis/action.

Though the diagnostic framework provided in **Table 2** presents a helpful mental model for classifying DSD diagnoses, the 'disorders' terminology contained within it (and used within the Consensus Statement more broadly) has been heavily critiqued. The terminology proposed in 2006 has largely been adopted by clinicians, but many affected individuals and their families prefer to use other terms, often due to the concern that the use of terms such as 'disorder' unnecessarily medicalizes normal human variation.[2] Some also distinguish the terms by describing DSD as a diagnosis and intersex as an identity.[3] Most commonly, affected individuals and their parents use the name of their specific condition.[4,5] Other terms have been proposed, including 'variations of sex characteristics', and 'conditions affecting reproductive development'.

In this review, we use 'DSD' as an abbreviation for 'differences of sex development', as a more objective description of the anatomy. Accordingly, we also use the term 'non-binary'[6] to describe external genital appearance that is not typically male or female (more commonly referred to as 'ambiguous' or 'atypical,' terms which may be stigmatizing). 'Intersex' is used in this review to describe an identity. Given that true consensus regarding terminology does not exist and further, that language is in constant evolution, clinicians and researchers should be cognizant of patient/family terminology preferences and be flexible in their use of terms.

Which Conditions Should Be Classified as Differences of Sex Development?

Just as DSD nomenclature is debatable, a lack of consensus exists on whether certain conditions should be classified under the DSD umbrella. Although there are potential psychosocial and research benefits from classifying a diverse range of chromosomal, gonadal, and anatomic conditions together, it is commonly questioned whether a DSD classification is appropriate for certain diagnoses (particularly CAH, proximal hypospadias, and certain sex chromosome disorders).

Many individuals with CAH (and their families) view the condition as an endocrine disorder rather than a DSD. A 2015 survey of CARES Foundation members reported multiple reasons for not preferring DSD terminology, including that DSD de-emphasizes the adrenal aspects of the condition, and the lack of difference in genital development among individuals with 46,XY karyotype and CAH due to 21-hydroxylase deficiency.[7] The CARES Foundation is a CAH advocacy and support organization, and, due to the concerns with nomenclature reported by many of their members, will not participate in studies that use DSD terminology. In another survey of patients and families accessing clinical care (not necessarily CARES Foundation members), individuals with CAH were more likely to use "just the diagnosis" to refer to their condition as compared to individuals with other DSD diagnoses.[5]

Table 1 Proposed revised nomenclature	
Previous	**Proposed**
Intersex	DSD
Male pseudohermaphrodite, undervirilization of an XY male, and undermasculinization of an XY male	46,XY DSD
Female pseudohermaphrodite, overvirilization of an XX female, and masculinization of an XX female	46,XX DSD
True hermaphrodite	Ovotesticular DSD
XX male or XX sex reversal	46,XX testicular DSD
XY sex reversal	46,XY complete gonadal dysgenesis

Table 2
An example of differences of sex development classification

Sex Chromosome DSD	46,XY DSD	46,XX DSD
45,X (Turner syndrome and variants)	*Disorders of gonadal (testicular) development*: (1) complete gonadal dysgenesis (Swyer syndrome); (2) partial gonadal dysgenesis; (3) gonadal regression; and (4) ovotesticular DSD	*Disorders of gonadal (ovarian) development*: (1) ovotesticular DSD; (2) testicular DSD (eg, SRY+duplicate SOX9); and (3) gonadal dysgenesis
47,XXY (Klinefelter syndrome and variants)	*Disorders in androgen synthesis or action*: (1) androgen biosynthesis defect (eg, 17-hydroxysteroid dehydrogenase deficiency, 5RD2 deficiency, StAR mutations); (2) defect in androgen action (eg, CAIS, PAIS); (3) luteinizing hormone receptor defects (eg, Leydig cell hypoplasia, aplasia); and (4) disorders of anti-Mullerian hormone and anti-Mullerian hormone receptor (persistent Mullerian duct syndrome)	*Androgen excess*: (1) fetal (eg, 21-hydroxylase deficiency, 11-hydroxylase deficiency); (2) fetoplacental (aromatase deficiency, POR [P450 Oxidoreductase]); and (3) maternal (luteoma, exogenous, etc.)
45,X/46,XY (MGD, ovotesticular DSD)		*Other* (eg, cloacal exstrophy, vaginal atresia, MURCS [Mullerian, renal, cervicothoracic somite abnormalities], other syndromes)
46,XX/46,XY (chimeric, ovotesticular DSD)		

There are differing opinions among pediatric urologists about whether all patients with proximal hypospadias should be considered to have "a DSD" or whether this label is best reserved for when a specific DSD diagnosis has been identified.[8] When interpreted literally, all patients with proximal hypospadias fit the 2006 consensus definition of DSD. However, many do not have a specific, identified known underlying etiology or genetic diagnosis. Practically, the DSD label is typically limited to those with proximal hypospadias with at least one undescended testis, as affirmed in the 2016 consensus update.[9] However, establishing a specific DSD diagnosis can be useful for discussing issues regarding gender and sex development, surgical counseling, future fertility, targeted psychosocial support, potential for gonadal tumor, and/or multisystem comorbidities (**Table 3**). Conversely, classifying a patient with proximal hypospadias with no specific identified cause as having a "46,XY DSD of unknown etiology" may contribute to social and legal controversy about the timing of hypospadias surgery, without many of the benefits of a specific DSD diagnosis.

Turner syndrome and Klinefelter syndrome are two sex chromosome differences that also do not neatly fall under the DSD umbrella. Both conditions are associated with impaired gonadal function, but not increased germ cell tumor risk

Table 3
Potential implications of differences of sex development diagnosis

Topic	Implication
Sex assignment/Future gender identity	• Can help inform sex assignment in infancy, based on gender identity data from adult populations (if available)
Surgical counseling	• Possible higher hypospadias surgical complication rates[10-12]
Fertility potential	• Predict fertility potential by DSD diagnosis • Determine eligibility for experimental gonadal tissue cryopreservation[13]
Hormonal function	• Proactive monitoring of hormone function for peer-concordant pubertal development, growth, bone health
Gonadal tumor risk	• Anticipatory guidance, screening, or gonadectomy for conditions in which there is a known gonadal tumor risk
Multisystem comorbidities	• Targeted screening for associated comorbidities
Genetic transmission	• Counseling about future pregnancies, possibility of transmission of condition to future offspring
Psychosocial health	• Community connections for peer support • Behavioral health professional support • Individual benefit of an explanation for genital difference

(except in cases of mosaic Turner syndrome with Y-chromosome) or non-binary genitalia. Many of the longitudinal health concerns encountered by patients with Turner syndrome and Klinefelter syndrome fall outside of the traditional DSD care team specialties. At our hospital, for example, there is a separate multidisciplinary clinic for patients with Turner syndrome, and we are currently developing a separate, similar clinic for patients with Klinefelter syndrome.

Multidisciplinary/Interdisciplinary Care Model

It is critical to be familiar with historical standards of DSD care to avoid perpetuating the harms of these standards in the current era in which our understanding of sex and gender development is expanding rapidly. Though a detailed discussion of historic trends is beyond the scope of this article, please see Witchel, and colleagues, 2022, for a recent review.[14] To summarize key points, prophylactic gonadectomy was historically strongly encouraged in cases where there was thought to be any potential for malignant transformation, or when the expected hormone and gamete production of the gonad did not align with the patient's sex assignment at birth. Non-binary genitalia was feared to cause gender identity "confusion" according to the prevailing notion of gender development at the time, so surgery on the external and/or internal genitalia was typically recommended in infancy. Age-appropriate disclosure of medical and surgical history to the patient and family was not routine. Notably, these historic trends in DSD care continue to directly influence current limitations in the field, with key examples being a lack of long-term data on tumor risk in intact gonads or on outcomes for patients who did not have early genital surgery.

A paradigm shift is now occurring in which bodily autonomy and shared decision-making ground management discussions. As such, a multidisciplinary approach becomes essential for nuanced, comprehensive care, with each specialty bringing an important perspective on diagnosis and management. As detailed below, the evolution of the diagnostic workup makes a clinician with genetics expertise invaluable. Surgical specialists (urologists, pediatric surgeons, gynecologists) and endocrinologists help frame complex discussions of options for hormonal manipulation, gonadal management, and surgical interventions. A behavioral health specialist provides support in clarifying the patient's and family's values and priorities that influence their decision-making. Patients and families benefit from access to ongoing professional mental and behavioral health support at different ages and stages, as well as informal peer support groups. There are also important roles for social workers, nurses, and health educators in patient and family support and education. Additional team members that may be called upon as needed include those providing fertility preservation or ethics consultation.

Advances in Diagnostic Testing/Evolution of the Diagnostic Evaluation

Several algorithms have been proposed for the evaluation of DSD, particularly for patients who have non-binary genitalia noted at birth, though there is little standardization.[15,16] Key components of this evaluation include early multidisciplinary collaboration, and carefully timed endocrine and genetic evaluation. Prenatal suspicion of DSD is also becoming more common, which is changing early conversations with many families. **Fig. 1** shows an approach to the newborn with a suspected DSD, emphasizing timing of elements of the evaluation and multidisciplinary collaboration. Typical investigations include measurement of adrenal and gonadal hormones, imaging of the gonads and reproductive structures, and genetic testing.[17] Several aspects of the evaluation are often in process concurrently; while awaiting karyotype results, multiple hormone tests may be sent, followed by genetic testing in a stepwise fashion over the course of many months. Occasionally, non-binary genital development is found to be due to prenatal hormone exposure or hormone disruptors, but a thorough history is usually sufficient to rule out these possibilities.

In-depth understanding of adrenal and gonadal physiology is needed to choose the relevant laboratory studies, as hormone production evolves rapidly over the first days and months of life, and even thereafter remains dependent on age/pubertal stage and time of day (circadian rhythm). Ultrasensitive or mass spectrometry based assays should be employed to detect potentially low levels of steroid hormones.[18,19] A dynamic test such as cosyntropin stimulation is low-risk and can rapidly provide reassurance of adequate cortisol production to allow safe hospital discharge for a neonate. More prolonged and intensive dynamic testing such as human chorionic gonadotropin stimulation may provide useful diagnostic information, but should be weighed against the potential harm of stimulating undesired androgen production as well as the burden to the patient and family of multiple injections and clinic visits.

Even with meticulous attention to detail, there are known pitfalls of relying on hormone levels for diagnosis of conditions affecting steroidogenesis or steroid action, including functional isoenzymes and backdoor pathways of steroidogenesis that can influence precursor-to-product ratios.[20–22]

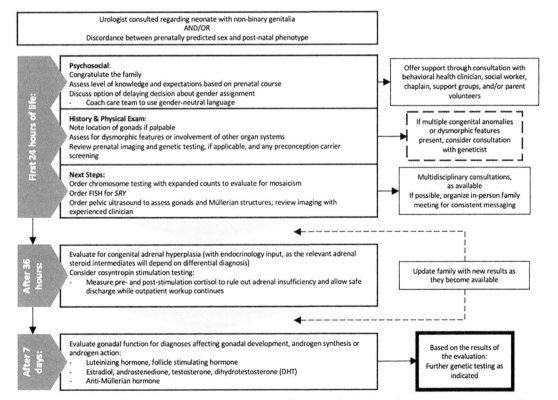

Fig. 1. Management of possible DSD in a neonate: Emphasis on the timing of workup and multidisciplinary collaboration. DSD, differences of sex development; FISH, fluorescence in situ hybridization; SRY, sex-determining region Y.

Further, a variety of DSD diagnoses may result in similar phenotypes and hormonal profiles that do not narrow the differential diagnosis substantially. For example, in a sample of patients with a phenotype of proximal hypospadias, various molecular genetic diagnoses were identified in 28%.[23] Thus, attempts to arrive at a specific genetic diagnosis are strongly recommended,[24] with benefits outlined in **Table 3**.

Single-gene sequencing may be prudent in cases where a diagnosis is suspected based on phenotype and chromosomal analysis, or a positive family history (eg, CAIS or 21-hydroxylase deficiency CAH). In other cases, concurrent sequencing of a large panel of genes known to affect reproductive development will be more comprehensive. The difficulty here arises as commercial gene panels become quickly outdated due to the discovery of new candidate genes. Whole-exome sequencing (WES) may have higher diagnostic yield[25,26] and may reduce the need for extensive hormonal testing.[27] WES offers the benefit of reanalysis at future time points to account for newly described genetic correlations. WES is expected to soon give way to whole genome sequencing (WGS) as cost continues to fall and availability expands.[28,29] WGS covers portions of the genome that are not analyzed by WES, including deep intronic regions, and it is able to provide a more accurate analysis of tandem repeats and paralogous regions than WES. Further, WGS can detect structural variants typically limited to detection by chromosomal microarray analysis (CMA), including copy number variants, insertions, inversions, and translocations. It has also been shown to have a higher diagnostic yield for a variety of indications than targeted gene panels and CMA technology.[30,31]

There is also an emerging evidence base for conceptualizing some DSDs as oligogenic (ie, where the phenotype is based on the effect of one gene/allele on a second gene/locus).[32] Many of the current diagnoses under the DSD umbrella, such as ovotesticular DSD or partial gonadal dysgenesis can more appropriately be thought of as umbrella terms themselves, encompassing a heterogeneous group of conditions with different outcomes in regard to hormone and gamete production, risk of gonadal tumor, and other organ system involvement.[33] We expect that as more patients learn a specific genetic diagnosis, we will be better able to stratify risk and thus management strategies.

DSD conditions that do not present with non-binary genitalia at birth were historically diagnosed due to precocious or delayed pubertal development, or development of secondary sex characteristics not expected based on sex assignment and presumed gonadal configuration at birth. Still other diagnoses may not be detected until adulthood (if ever) due to subfertility or infertility. This diagnostic timing pattern is changing with the introduction and proliferation of cell-free fetal DNA (cfDNA) screening technology in which fragments of fetal DNA are isolated from peripheral blood of the gestational parent to predict fetal sex (with the stated goal of screening for chromosomal aneuploidies, deletions, and duplications).[34,35] Here, also, much work has been done to lay out diagnostic algorithms for cases of non-binary genitalia on prenatal ultrasound, or discordance between expected karyotype based on cfDNA and the reproductive phenotype observed on ultrasound or postnatal physical examination.[36–38] Conditions incidentally diagnosed prenatally in this way may include 46,XX testicular DSD due to SRY translocation or 46,XY complete gonadal dysgenesis.

Over time, we expect that earlier and more comprehensive detection will change the demographics of the affected populations and allow improved predictions of risk of complications and other outcomes, rather than relying on data extrapolated from the limited population seeking medical attention due to symptomatology.

Sex Assignment at Birth and Future Gender Identity

Gender identity development is not well understood, and future gender identity cannot be predicted for any infant with absolute certainty. In many categories of DSD, there appears to be a higher rate of identification as a gender other than that aligned with the sex assigned at birth, even with diligent diagnostics to guide initial sex assignment.[39,40] Compiling reliable data on adult gender identity for specific DSD diagnoses is very challenging. First, the social and cultural factors that influence the conceptualization of sex, gender identity, gender roles, and gender expression have varied over time and around the world and impact how patient outcome data are reported in the literature[41] (such as recording the patient's observed gender expression or social gender role rather than directly inquiring about gender identity or concept of self). In many parts of the world, the sociocultural landscape is changing rapidly, with intersex, transgender, and non-binary identities becoming more visible and accepted.[42] Individuals who may have felt the risk of stigma or discrimination was previously too great may now feel able to publicly identify themselves or now feel they have an accurate language to describe their identities. There has also been a greater tendency to assign a male sex to infants with non-binary genitalia over the last several decades, though the outcome of this trend is uncertain since for many of those patients, their adult gender identity has not yet been reported.[43]

The diagnosis of a newborn with DSD is often framed as a social emergency necessitating rapid evaluation for the purpose of assigning a sex of rearing. Families also frequently recall experiencing a sense of shock and lack of familiarity from health care providers when their child with a DSD was born. Thus, our program has emphasized the need for expedient multidisciplinary care for families who experience the newborn period as highly traumatic. Our patients' experiences highlight the essential need for the involvement of different specialists other than endocrinologists and urologists, as psychoeducation around the biological complexities of sex development and the frequency of identifying variations in sex development can provide context and reassurance for families. Reframing the conversation to acknowledge the inherent uncertainty in sex assignment for every infant can also be helpful. There is no diagnostic test to determine gender identity other than to ask the individual to describe their gender themselves when they are old enough to do so. Sex assignment and potential future gender identity should be discussed with families as soon as it is recognized that the child may have a DSD. However, this should be framed as a statement of the limitations of our ability to predict or influence gender identity development rather than providing a "warning" that their child may experience incongruence between their assigned sex and their gender identity. The team can also suggest strategies to support the child's self-expression and instill appreciation for diversity. Again, the support of a behavioral health professional with training in gender development can guide families toward an openness about their child's future[44] —drawing from the literature on transgender youth, parental acceptance has been shown to contribute to improved psychosocial adjustment.[45] **Box 1** provides tips for counseling families of infants born with a suspected DSD.

Gonadal Management

As mentioned above, gonadectomy was historically an automatic recommendation for any patient with a DSD with an increased risk of gonadal malignancy. Over the last several decades, understanding of gonadal tumor risk by diagnosis and

---

> **Box 1**
> **Counseling regarding sex assignment in infancy**
>
> 1. *Congratulate the family* on the birth of the infant.
> 2. *Inquire about the expected sex of the infant* based on prenatal testing, and whether an announcement about name and sex designation has been made to family/friends.
> 3. If such an announcement has been made, *use the name and pronouns that the family is using* for the baby.
> 4. Otherwise, *use gender-neutral terminology* (eg, 'the baby,' 'your baby,' and pronouns they/them/theirs). *Never use the pronoun 'it'.*
> 5. Lay groundwork for understanding differences in sex development by describing typical male and female sex development pathways, adjusting explanation as needed to the level of health literacy of the family.
> 6. Describe the infant's anatomy to the family using neutral terminology (eg, labioscrotal folds, gonads), pointing out how their development may have differed from typical pathways.
> 7. Discuss timeline for recommended diagnostic workup and *provide option to delay naming and sex assignment* until more diagnostic information is known.
> 8. Avoid framing our inability to predict future gender identity with certainty as a potential problem or "risk"—*normalize gender diversity.*
> 9. *Provide psychosocial support* through formal consultations with behavioral health providers and/or parent/support group connections.

---

age has advanced to allow more individualized counseling and decision-making.[46–48] As one example, the overall risk of gonadal tumors among individuals with CAIS is thought to be low (<10% in most studies),[48–50] and the development of tumors before puberty is rare. Also, patients with CAIS experience endogenous puberty due to peripheral aromatization of testosterone to estrogen and have ongoing hormonal production. Therefore, it is becoming common for these individuals to retain their gonads at least until linear growth is complete. At that age, the patient is usually able to participate in a shared decision-making approach regarding the risk of tumor development. A management protocol was suggested by Weidler and colleagues in 2019.[50]

In the past, fertility potential was not thought to be possible for many DSD conditions. This assumption is also being reconsidered, and experimental gonadal tissue cryopreservation is now being offered at some centers for patients with DSD who have elected for prophylactic gonadectomy due to tumor risk.[13,51] Advances in assisted reproductive technology will be necessary for gonadal tissue cryopreserved from individuals with DSD to be used to produce a biological child in the future. However, promising progress in prepubertal ovarian and testicular tissue maturation is occurring,[52,53] and these advances may ultimately extend to the gonadal tissue of patients with DSD. As genetic testing and the ability to follow individuals by genetic diagnosis improve, we anticipate an increasingly personalized assessment of true fertility potential and tumor risk. These anticipated advances will improve our ability to counsel families about how strongly to consider gonadectomy at different ages.

Role of and Evolution of External Genital Surgery

External genital surgery for individuals with DSD has evolved significantly in the past 20 years. Controversy exists regarding many aspects of DSD surgery, most notably the timing of surgical procedures, outcomes assessment, and terminology. In the broadest sense, external genital surgery has traditionally been divided into feminizing and masculinizing procedures, though there is controversy about whether 'feminizing' and 'masculinizing' are the most appropriate terms. This review recognizes this controversy but utilizes these terms since alternative and updated terms are not yet available. The evolution of feminizing and masculinizing surgical approaches will be discussed and the controversy of the timing of surgery will also be examined.

In feminizing surgery, there are three separate components: clitoroplasty, vaginoplasty, and labioplasty. These can be done in combination in one stage or performed separately. Collectively, when done in one stage, the procedures are commonly referred to as 'feminizing genitoplasty'. Improvements in functional and cosmetic outcomes of feminizing genitoplasty have largely been due to the experience gained in patients with CAH, the most common group of patients who are candidates for this surgery. Regarding clitoroplasty, we previously evolved from performing clitoral reduction/resection (no longer done) to clitoral recession. More recently, further elucidation of the innervation of the clitoris has resulted in the development of the modern nerve-sparing clitoroplasty.[54–56] This allows for a reduction in the size of the clitoris while maintaining the neurovascular bundles and innervation of the glans clitoris. Long-term studies that have been performed thus far have demonstrated that clitoral sensation and function appear to be adequately preserved with nerve-sparing clitoroplasty[57] although further functional studies in adults are still needed.

The ability to address the persistent urogenital sinus in patients with CAH and other forms of DSD has also evolved significantly. Traditionally, a perineal-based skin flap vaginoplasty was performed in cases where the vagina had a low takeoff from the common urogenital sinus channel. When a high takeoff of the vagina is present, separation of the vagina from the common channel is needed, given that a skin flap cannot reach the posterior wall of the vagina. Separation of the vagina from the common channel can be technically challenging since the posterior aspect of the urethra and anterior vagina are partially fused and often share a common wall. Thus, separation can result in deficiency in one or both walls. Hence, significant postoperative complications can occur including urethrovaginal fistula formation and stenosis of the reconstructed urethra and/or vagina. The surgical technique for vaginoplasty has been revolutionized with the development of total urogenital sinus mobilization (TUM). This technique was originally described by Pena and colleagues[58] in patients with persistent cloaca and anorectal malformations and has now been successfully applied to patients with CAH. TUM allows for mobilization of the entire urogenital sinus as a unit without formally separating the vagina from the common channel. With distal mobilization of the sinus, separate openings for the urethra and vagina can be achieved without the need to separate the vagina. However, certain patients may develop urinary incontinence following TUM, especially those with a short urethra.[59] Thus, Rink and colleagues, have modified this technique where deep dissection is limited to the posterior and lateral aspects of the urogenital sinus while attempting to better preserve the anterior bladder neck competence mechanism (partial urogenital sinus mobilization, PUM).[60] In cases of a long common channel and high takeoff of the vagina, separation of the vagina may still be needed. Surgical exposure to facilitate this difficult dissection is a challenge although improvements have been made with the perineal prone technique[61] and anterior sagittal transrectal approaches.[62] Lastly, refinements in labioplasty and modified use of the common urogenital sinus tissue have allowed for a more anatomically female-typical configuration of the vaginal introitus, labia minora, and labia majora.[56]

Masculinizing surgery in patients with DSD is in most cases identical to surgery for proximal (peno-scrotal or perineal) hypospadias. As is the case with feminizing genitoplasty, this surgery has evolved significantly although it is still one that is associated with a high complication rate and in need of further improvement.[63] Studies from high-volume centers demonstrate that the long-term results of traditional proximal hypospadias procedures have a high complication rate, regardless of whether the repair is done in one or two stages.[64–66] Recurrent chordee and/or urethral complications can exceed 50% when patients are followed through adolescence. Preliminary data from a prospective multi-institutional study in patients with 46,XY DSD show a similar high complication rate following masculinizing surgery.[67] In general, one-stage techniques have now fallen out of favor. Most experts agree that a two-stage repair will achieve the best functional and cosmetic results in which the urethral plate is divided and the chordee is corrected at the time of the first stage. Ventral approaches to correct the chordee (corporal body grafting, deep transverse incisions of the tunica albuginea, and full-thickness corporotomies) are more successful than dorsal plication in straightening the penis but may have an increased incidence of erectile dysfunction later in life.[68] Second-stage urethroplasty is best accomplished with free grafts of preputial skin or modified combination flap/grafts.[69–71] Traditional use of Byar's flaps as the tissue that will be tubularized in the second stage should be avoided.

The timing of external genital surgery is currently under tremendous scrutiny. Decades ago, early surgery was advocated with the philosophy that patients tolerate surgery better as infants, have no recollection of the surgery, and have improved results compared to patients who have surgery at an older age. Based on the philosophy of John Money,[72] it was also felt that patients uniformly did well from a psychosocial standpoint with early sex assignment and surgery to align the anatomy with that sex assignment. It is now known that this philosophy is incorrect and that many individuals will declare later in life that their gender identity is incongruent with their sex assigned at birth. In such individuals, early irreversible surgery (ie, clitoral reduction) can potentially be catastrophic. Further, there may be regret among adults who had surgery as young children due to surgical complications, or lack of involvement of the individual in the decision to have genital surgery. Thus, the current recommended approaches are

for open and transparent discussions with families regarding the risks and benefits of early versus late surgery that occur at a multidisciplinary center with input from numerous specialists. Ideally, irreversible forms of genital surgery should be avoided until the individual can adequately participate in this decision-making process. The exact age of when this is possible will vary depending on the individual and their condition. In cases of surgical decision-making by caregivers in infancy and childhood, an understanding of the limitations of our ability to predict a child's gender identity, future embodiment goals, or fertility desires is an essential component of thorough informed consent.

As discussed, certain DSD conditions are associated with a higher rate of identification as a gender other than that aligned with the sex assigned at birth, and here, there is general agreement that avoiding irreversible surgery in infancy is appropriate. However, in certain populations like 46,XX patients with CAH, the role of early surgery is less clear.[73,74] The majority of available literature indicates that most patients with CAH and their parents support access to early surgery.[75,76] However, there is an increased incidence of male gender identity in these patients[77] (who may prefer no surgery, or desire masculinizing genitoplasty). It also cannot be assumed that all who identify as female want a female-typical external genital appearance or would be willing to accept the risks of surgery to achieve this. These scenarios present several instances in which irreversible clitoral surgery may be performed as an infant when the patient themselves would have preferred that tissue be maintained. Therefore, it is now being questioned whether it is appropriate to perform feminizing genitoplasty in infancy, even when the families are educated on all the controversial aspects of early surgery and its potential complications. What is sorely lacking in this debate is knowledge of the natural history and psychosocial status of patients who do not have early surgery. Until more knowledge is gained regarding the long-term results and consequences in patients who do and do not have surgery, physicians need to be very transparent about the controversies that exist when counseling families of infants with CAH regarding early surgery.

Advocacy, Activism, and Relationship with the Medical Community

Advocacy groups, peer support groups, and the medical community all desire to better define and deliver excellent, high-quality care for patients with DSD and their families. Over the last two decades, the relationship between these groups has become more polarized in many parts of the world, especially in the United States. This is in part due to the perception from many advocacy and activism groups that the medical community has not adequately involved them in discussions that help to define the standard of care for intersex individuals, as well as concerns that their voices are not being adequately represented. Many intersex advocates assert that any genital surgery in patients with DSD performed without their assent that is not medically necessary is considered a human rights violation. This viewpoint was formalized in the joint report from InterACT and the Human Rights Watch entitled "I Want to be Like Nature Made Me".[78] This perspective about early genital surgery has also been supported by the World Health Organization,[79] the United Nations[80] (REF), and three former US Surgeons General.[81] Some advocacy groups have proposed legislation that institutes a blanket moratorium on genital surgery in infants with DSD, the language of which may be interpreted to extend to more routine urologic procedures such as orchidopexies or circumcisions. Most physicians do not favor such a broad moratorium, arguing that individuals with DSD represent a very diverse group of patients, and it is not possible to make a blanket statement on the role of surgery that will benefit all patients. There is also the concern that such an approach would inappropriately interfere with the patient–physician relationship.

Ideally, advocacy groups and the medical community should work together and engage in nuanced conversations to achieve progress toward individualized care of the highest quality for patients with DSD. Despite the differences of opinion that exist between many advocates and many in the medical community, there are several recommendations that we believe should receive broad support. It is abundantly clear that the medical community needs to better seek out the opinion of their patients on which outcomes are most important to them, and to encourage patients and their families to speak with advocacy and peer support groups. There needs to be complete transparency in the discussion of previous medical and surgical approaches that are no longer recommended, and a willingness to accept critique of past treatments. An honest and self-reflective approach of the medical community plus increased transparency will hopefully lead to more productive conversations with advocacy groups and a renewed level of trust.

Additionally, an issue that requires better clarity is whether the opinions expressed by advocacy groups represent the majority viewpoint of individuals with DSD or whether there is a large, less vocal, group whose views are not being represented. Many patients desire to maintain privacy regarding their DSD diagnosis, making this difficult to discern, but some data are being accrued to help in this effort. In a multi-center survey from Europe, over 450 adult patients with varying DSD diagnoses were queried on their personal views regarding early surgery. Thirteen percent of those surveyed felt that they would have been better off without early surgery, and "participant perspectives varied considerably by diagnostic category, gender, history of surgery, and contact with support groups." The authors concluded that "outcome data failed to support a general moratorium on early elective genital surgery" and noted that "case-by-case decision-making is better suited to grasping the ethical complexity of the issues at stake".[75]

Early surgery aside, the many other ways in which a DSD diagnosis may impact an individual across the lifespan are vastly understudied. Additional research is needed on topics including, but not limited to, clarifying the true risk of gonadal tumors in different diagnoses, optimizing hormone replacement regimens for bone and cardiovascular health, and improving fertility preservation or restoration for those who desire it.

Lastly, there is a need to create a different narrative in the public eye by clearly defining our current level of knowledge and where gaps exist. We need to acknowledge current deficiencies in evidence-based research and explain that our current decision-making process is based on the best available evidence. We can then take concrete steps toward filling in knowledge gaps with sound scientific investigations. Input from the intersex community should be sought throughout the research process. It is our hope that the relationship between advocacy and activism groups and the medical community can move from an adversarial stance toward one promoting positive and beneficial change in the coming years.

SUMMARY

DSD diagnoses encompass a wide range of conditions that require a multidisciplinary approach, and we advocate for this care model for all individuals with DSD. Diagnosis and management of DSD has evolved substantially over the last several decades and continues. There are many unanswered questions that require further research and collaboration between patients, families, advocates, and medical professionals.

CLINICS CARE POINTS

- Many aspects of DSD care are evolving and controversial, underscoring the importance of a multidisciplinary approach.
- Given the lack of agreement about DSD terminology, clinicians should remain flexible about nomenclature including asking patients and families which terms they would like to use.
- Algorithms are available to guide both prenatal and postnatal evaluation of suspected DSD.
- Advanced genetic testing options (eg, whole exome and WGS) have now been expanded to patients with suspected DSD, and have the potential to simplify the diagnostic process.
- Individuals with some DSD conditions appear to have a higher rate of gender identification that is different than the sex assigned at birth. Early and regular mental and behavioral health involvement helps to support families as they learn about sex and gender development, and their child's specific diagnosis.
- Prophylactic gonadectomy is no longer an automatic recommendation for patients with DSD conditions that confer an increased risk of gonadal tumors. The current approach to gonadal management includes an individualized shared decision-making process that incorporates diagnosis, age, expected hormonal and fertility potential, and patient/family goals.
- Urologists should maintain an appreciation for different perspectives on the type and timing of external genital surgery. These differing perspectives, and knowns and unknowns about surgical outcomes, should be shared with families as part of the shared decision-making process about whether to perform external genital surgery, and if so, timing and type.

DISCLOSURE

All authors declare no disclosures/conflicts of interest related to this work.

ACKNOWLEDGMENTS

The authors acknowledge Elizabeth Leeth, MS, CGC and Allison Weisman, MS, CGC for their review of and contributions to the genetics-related content within this article.

REFERENCES

1. Lee PA, Houk CP, Ahmed SF, et al. International Consensus Conference on Intersex organized by the Lawson Wilkins Pediatric Endocrine S, the European Society for Paediatric E. Consensus statement on management of intersex disorders. International Consensus Conference on Intersex. Pediatrics 2006;118(2):e488–500.
2. Reis E. Divergence or disorder?: the politics of naming intersex. Perspect Biol Med 2007;50(4):535–43.
3. Johnson EK, Rosoklija I, Finlayson C, et al. Attitudes towards "disorders of sex development" nomenclature among affected individuals. J Pediatr Urol 2017;13(6):e601–8.
4. Tiryaki S, Tekin A, Yagmur İ, et al. Parental Perception of Terminology of Disorders of Sex Development in Western Turkey. J Clin Res Pediatr Endocrinol 2018;10(3):216–22.
5. D'Oro A, Rosoklija I, Jacobson DL, et al. Patient and Caregiver Attitudes toward Disorders of Sex Development Nomenclature. J Urol 2020;204(4):835–42.
6. Pyle LC. Origin of non-binary genitalia. Personal email communication to J Whitehead 2022.
7. Lin-Su K, Lekarev O, Poppas DP, et al. Congenital adrenal hyperplasia patient perception of 'disorders of sex development' nomenclature. Int J Pediatr Endocrinol 2015;2015(1):9.
8. Snodgrass W, Macedo A, Hoebeke P, et al. Hypospadias dilemmas: a round table. J Pediatr Urol 2011;7(2):145–57.
9. Lee PA, Nordenstrom A, Houk CP, et al. Global Disorders of Sex Development Update since 2006: Perceptions, Approach and Care. Horm Res Paediatr 2016;85(3):158–80.
10. Saltzman AF, Carrasco A Jr, Colvin A, et al. Patients with disorders of sex development and proximal hypospadias are at high risk for reoperation. World J Urol 2018;36(12):2051–8.
11. Ochi T, Ishiyama A, Yazaki Y, et al. Surgical management of hypospadias in cases with concomitant disorders of sex development. Pediatr Surg Int 2019;35(5):611–7.
12. Palmer BW, Reiner W, Kropp BP. Proximal hypospadias repair outcomes in patients with a specific disorder of sexual development diagnosis. Adv Urol 2012;2012:708301.
13. Johnson EK, Finlayson C, Finney EL, et al. Gonadal tissue cryopreservation for children with differences of sex development. Horm Res Paediatr 2019;92(2):84–91.
14. Witchel S, Mazur T, Houk C, et al. The long path to our current understanding regarding care of children with differences/disorders of sexual

development. Hormone Research in Pediatrics 2022;95:608–18.

15. Committee on Genetics, Section on Urology, Section on Endocrinology. Evaluation of the newborn with developmental anomalies of the external genitalia. Pediatrics 2000;106(1):138–42.

16. Leon N, Reyes A, Harley V. A clinical algorithm to diagnose differences of sex development. Lancet Diabetes Endocrinol 2019;February:1–15.

17. O'Connell MA, Atlas G, Ayers K, et al. Establishing a molecular genetic diagnosis in children with Differences of Sex Development - a clinical approach. Horm Res Paediatr 2021. https://doi.org/10.1159/000520926.

18. Rosner W, Hankinson S, Sluss P, et al. Challenges to the measurement of estradiol: an Endocrine Society position statement. Journal Clin Endocrinol Metab 2013;98(4):1376–87.

19. Courant F, Aksglaede L, Antignac J-P, et al. Assessment of circulating sex steroid levels in prepubertal and pubertal boys and girls by a novel ultrasensitive gas chromatography-tandem mass spectrometry method. Journal Clin Endocrinol Metab 2010;95(1):82–92.

20. Ahmed SF, Iqbal A, Hughes I. The testosterone:androstenedione ratio in male undermasculinization. Clin Endocrinol 2000;53:697–702.

21. Khattab A, Yuen T, Yau M, et al. Pitfalls in hormonal diagnosis of 17-beta hydroxysteroid dehydrogenase III deficiency. J Pediatr Endocr Met 2015;28(5–6):623–8.

22. Miller W, Auchus R. The "backdoor pathway" of androgen synthesis in human male sexual development. PLoS Biol 2019;17(4):1–6.

23. Johnson EK, Jacobson D, Finlayson C, et al. Proximal hypospadias - isolated genital condition or marker of more? J Urol 2020;204(2):345–52.

24. Cools M, Nordenstrom A, Robeva R, et al. Caring for individuals with a difference of sex development (DSD): a consensus statement. Nat Rev Endocrinol 2018;14(7):415–29.

25. Gomes NL, Batista RL, Nishi MY, et al. Contribution of clinical and genetic approaches for diagnosing 209 index cases with 46,XY differences of sex development. J Clin Endocrinol Metab 2022;107:e1797–806.

26. Xie QG, Luo P, Xia K, et al. 46,XY disorders of sex development: the use of NGS for prevalent variants. Hum Genet 2022;141(12):1863–73.

27. Tenenbaum Rakover Y., Admoni O., Assad G.E., et al., Novel genes involved in sex differentiation identified by whole-exome sequencing in a cohort of children with disorders of sex development [Abstract], Journal of the Endocrine Society, 4 (Suppl 1), 2020. PMCID: PMC7208792.

28. French C, Delon I, Dolling H, et al. Whole genome sequencing reveals that genetic conditions are frequent in intensively ill children. Intensive Care Med 2019;45(5):627–36.

29. Bick D, Jones M, Taylor S, et al. Case for genome sequencing in infants and children with rare, undiagnosed or genetic diseases. J Med Genet 2019;56(12):783–91.

30. Stavropoulos DJ, Merico D, Jobling R, et al. Whole Genome Sequencing Expands Diagnostic Utility and Improves Clinical Management in Pediatric Medicine. NPJ Genom Med 2016;1:15012.

31. Parivesh A, Barseghyan H, Delot E, et al. Translating genomics to the clinical diagnosis of disorders/differences of sex development. Curr Top Dev Biol 2019;134:317–75.

32. Camats N, Flueck C, Audi L. Oligogenic origin of differences of sex development in humans. Int J Mol Sci 2020;21(1809):1–14.

33. Syryn H, Van De Vijver K, Cools M. Ovotesticular Difference of Sex Development: Genetic Background, Histological Features, and Clinical Management. Horm Res Paediatr 2021. https://doi.org/10.1159/000519323.

34. Gregg A, Skotko B, Benkendorf J, et al. Noninvasive prenatal screening for fetal aneuploidy, 2016 update: a position statement of the American College of Medical Genetics and Genomics. Genet Med 2016;18(10):1056–65.

35. Committee on Practice Bulletins. Screening for fetal chromosomal abnormalities: ACOG Practice Bulletin. Obstet Gynecol 2020;136(4):e48–69.

36. Chitty L, Chatelain P, Wolffenbuttel K, et al. Prenatal management of disorders of sex development. J Pediatr Urol 2012;8:576–84.

37. Chitayat D, Glanc P. Diagnostic approach in prenatally detected genital abnormalities. Ultrasound Obstet Gynecol 2010;35:637–46.

38. Byers H, Neufeld-Kaiser W, Chang E, et al. Discordant sex between fetal screening and postnatal phenotype requires evaluation. J Perinatol 2019;39:28–33.

39. Bakula D, Mullins A, Sharkey C, et al. Gender identity outcomes in children with disorders/differences of sex development: predictive factors. Semin Perinatol 2017;17:214–7.

40. de Vries A, Doreleijers T, Cohen-Kettenis P. Disorders of sex development and gender identity outcome in adolescence and adulthood: understanding gender identity development and its clinical implications. Pediatr Endocrinol Rev 2007;4(4):343–51.

41. Weidler E, Peterson K. The impact of culture on disclosure in differences of sex development. Semin Pediatr Surg 2019;28:1–5.

42. Parker K, Menasce Horowitz J, Brown A. Americans' Complex Views on Gender Identity and Transgender Issues. Available at: https://www.pewresearch.org/social-trends/2022/06/28/americans-complex-views-on-gender-identity-and-transgender-issues/. Published 2022. Accessed January 25, 2023.

43. Kolesinska Z, Ahmed F, Niedziela M, et al. Changes over time in sex assignment for disorders of sex development. Pediatrics 2014;134(3):e710–5.

44. van de Grift T. Condition openness is associated with better mental health in individuals with an intersex/differences of sex development condition: structural equation modeling of European multicenter data. Psychol Med 2021;53(6):1–12.

45. Olson K, Durwood L, DeMeules M, et al. Mental health of transgender children who are supported in their identities. Pediatrics 2016;137(3):1–8.

46. Looijenga LH, Hersmus R, Oosterhuis JW, et al. Tumor risk in disorders of sex development (DSD). Best Pract Res Clin Endocrinol Metabol 2007; 21(3):480–95.

47. Looijenga LH, Hersmus R, de Leeuw BH, et al. Gonadal tumours and DSD. Best Pract Res Clin Endocrinol Metabol 2010;24(2):291–310.

48. Slowikowska-Hilczer J, Szarras-Czapnik M, Duranteau L, et al. Risk of gonadal neoplasia in patients with disorders/differences of sex development. Cancer Epidemiol 2020;69:101800.

49. Hannema SE, Scott IS, Rajpert-De Meyts E, et al. Testicular development in the complete androgen insensitivity syndrome. J Pathol 2006;208(4): 518–27.

50. Weidler EM, Linnaus ME, Baratz AB, et al. A Management Protocol for Gonad Preservation in Patients with Androgen Insensitivity Syndrome. J Pediatr Adolesc Gynecol 2019;32(6):605–11.

51. Harris CJ, Corkum KS, Finlayson C, et al. Establishing an Institutional Gonadal Tissue Cryopreservation Protocol for Patients with Differences of Sex Development. J Urol 2020;204(5):1054–61.

52. Demeestere I, Simon P, Dedeken L, et al. Live birth after autograft of ovarian tissue cryopreserved during childhood. Hum Reprod 2015;30(9):2107–9.

53. Fayomi AP, Peters K, Sukhwani M, et al. Autologous grafting of cryopreserved prepubertal rhesus testis produces sperm and offspring. Science 2019; 363(6433):1314–9.

54. Baskin LS, Erol A, Li YW, et al. Anatomical studies of the human clitoris. J Urol 1999;162(3 Pt 2): 1015–20.

55. Poppas DP, Hochsztein AA, Baergen RN, et al. Nerve sparing ventral clitoroplasty preserves dorsal nerves in congenital adrenal hyperplasia. J Urol 2007;178(4 Pt 2):1802–6. discussion 1806.

56. Leslie JA, Cain MP, Rink RC. Feminizing genital reconstruction in congenital adrenal hyperplasia. Indian J Urol 2009;25(1):17–26.

57. Yang J, Felsen D, Poppas DP. Nerve sparing ventral clitoroplasty: analysis of clitoral sensitivity and viability. J Urol 2007;178(4 Pt 2):1598–601.

58. Pena A, Levitt MA, Hong A, et al. Surgical management of cloacal malformations: a review of 339 patients. J Pediatr Surg 2004;39(3):470–9. discussion 470-479.

59. Stites J, Bernabe KJ, Galan D, et al. Urinary continence outcomes following vaginoplasty in patients with congenital adrenal hyperplasia. J Pediatr Urol 2017;13(1):38 e31–e38 e37.

60. Rink RC, Metcalfe PD, Kaefer MA, et al. Partial urogenital mobilization: a limited proximal dissection. J Pediatr Urol 2006;2(4):351–6.

61. Rink RC, Pope JC, Kropp BP, et al. Reconstruction of the high urogenital sinus: early perineal prone approach without division of the rectum. J Urol 1997;158(3 Pt 2):1293–7.

62. Salle JL, Lorenzo AJ, Jesus LE, et al. Surgical treatment of high urogenital sinuses using the anterior sagittal transrectal approach: a useful strategy to optimize exposure and outcomes. J Urol 2012; 187(3):1024–31.

63. Gong EM, Cheng EY. Current challenges with proximal hypospadias: We have a long way to go. J Pediatr Urol 2017;13(5):457–67.

64. Stanasel I, Le HK, Bilgutay A, et al. Complications following Staged Hypospadias Repair Using Transposed Preputial Skin Flaps. J Urol 2015;194(2): 512–6.

65. McNamara ER, Schaeffer AJ, Logvinenko T, et al. Management of Proximal Hypospadias with 2-Stage Repair: 20-Year Experience. J Urol 2015;194(4): 1080–5.

66. Long CJ, Chu DI, Tenney RW, et al. Intermediate-Term Followup of Proximal Hypospadias Repair Reveals High Complication Rate. J Urol 2017;197(3 Pt 2):852–8.

67. Long CJ, Van Batavia J, Wisniewski AB, et al. Postoperative complications following masculinizing genitoplasty in moderate to severe genital atypia: results from a multicenter, observational prospective cohort study. J Pediatr Urol 2021;17(3): 379–86.

68. Husmann DA. Erectile dysfunction in patients undergoing multiple attempts at hypospadias repair: Etiologies and concerns. J Pediatr Urol 2021;17(2): e161–7.

69. Snodgrass W, Bush N. Staged Tubularized Autograft Repair for Primary Proximal Hypospadias with 30-Degree or Greater Ventral Curvature. J Urol 2017; 198(3):680–6.

70. Pippi Salle JL, Sayed S, Salle A, et al. Proximal hypospadias: A persistent challenge. Single institution outcome analysis of three surgical techniques over a 10-year period. J Pediatr Urol 2016;12(1): e21–7.

71. Chan YY, D'Oro A, Yerkes EB, et al. Challenging proximal hypospadias repairs: An evolution of technique for two stage repairs. J Pediatr Urol 2021; 17(2):e221–8.

72. Money J. Ablatio penis: normal male infant sex-reassigned as a girl. Arch Sex Behav 1975;4(1):65–71.

73. Binet A, Lardy H, Geslin D, et al. Should we question early feminizing genitoplasty for patients with congenital adrenal hyperplasia and XX karyotype? J Pediatr Surg 2016;51(3):465–8.

74. Szymanski KM, Whittam B, Kaefer M, et al. Parental decisional regret and views about optimal timing of female genital restoration surgery in congenital adrenal hyperplasia. J Pediatr Urol 2018;14(2):e151–7.

75. Bennecke E, Bernstein S, Lee P, et al. Early Genital Surgery in Disorders/Differences of Sex Development: Patients' Perspectives. Arch Sex Behav 2021;50(3):913–23.

76. Meyer-Bahlburg HFL. The Timing of Genital Surgery in Somatic Intersexuality: Surveys of Patients' Preferences. Horm Res Paediatr 2022;95(1):12–20.

77. de Jesus LE, Costa EC, Dekermacher S. Gender dysphoria and XX congenital adrenal hyperplasia: how frequent is it? Is male-sex rearing a good idea? J Pediatr Surg 2019;54(11):2421–7.

78. InterACT, Human Rights Watch (Organization). "I want to be like nature made me":medically unnecessary surgeries on intersex children in the US. Amsterdam: Human Rights Watch; 2017.

79. World Health Organization. Sexual health, human rights and the law. Geneva: World Health Organization; 2015.

80. Intersex people: OHCHR and the human rights of LGBTI people. Available at: https://www.ohchr.org/en/sexual-orientation-and-gender-identity/intersex-people. Published 2023. Accessed March 8, 2023.

81. Elders MJ, Satcher D, Carmona R. Re-Thinking Genital Surgeries on Intersex Infants. Available at: https://palmcenterlegacy.org/publication/re-thinking-genital-surgeries-intersex-infants/. Published 2017. Accessed March 8, 2023.

What Adults Teach Urologists About Hypospadias

Warren Snodgrass, MD*, Nicol Bush, MD, MCS

KEYWORDS

• Adult hypospadias • Urine spraying • Penile curvature • Sexual dysfunction

KEY POINTS

- Men with hypospadias who have no glans fusion have increased risk for urine spraying.
- As many as one of every three men with uncorrected distal hypospadias have penile curvature which can impact sexual function.
- Hypospadias repair can be done in adults with the same expected outcomes as in boys, but the overall experience for them is more traumatic.
- The consequences of uncorrected, or unsuccessfully corrected, hypospadias can impact a man's well-being throughout life.

Hypospadias occurs in one of every 200 males, of which most are distal with the meatus located somewhere on the distal penile shaft to the proximal glans. Today, these boys can have their penis made normal with a high likelihood of success and low risk for complications by tubularized incised plate (TIP) repair. In contrast to earlier times, this operation can be used for all variations in distal meatal location and anatomy. The only contraindication is ventral penile curvature that persists after degloving and measures 30° or more.[1]

Despite this, some question if distal hypospadias requires repair, and how that decision should be made. One obvious question is the consequences of uncorrected hypospadias in adults, but pediatric urologists who repair most hypospadias typically do not treat adults, whereas general and adult reconstructive urologists do not often encounter men with hypospadias. Yet, men with uncorrected, or unsuccessfully corrected, hypospadias have important lessons to teach all urologists. Those include that abnormal anatomy causes abnormal function. Ventral penile curvature causes sexual dysfunction for both men and their lovers. The appearance of the penis matters.

Taken together, we can summarize that boys with hypospadias grow into men who want a normal penis.

Earlier reports painted a different picture. One said that one of every 10 men they considered normal had a proximal glanular meatus yet described satisfactory function and that men with a coronal or subcoronal meatus were often unaware their penis was different.[2] Another agreed that a third of men they reviewed with distal hypospadias did not know they had the condition and that others who had a spraying or deflected stream or "mild to moderate" ventral curvature were not interested in surgery—which led them to conclude that men with hypospadias grow accustomed to their situation over time.[3]

Recent studies draw different conclusions. A survey of men self-identified with distal hypospadias found that they were less satisfied than normal men with the shape and position of their meatus and reported more ventral curvature and difficulties with sexual intercourse.[4] A second stated that six of seven men with uncorrected hypospadias had difficulties voiding,[5] whereas a third reviewing men referred by general urologists

Hypospadias Specialty Center, 3716 Standridge Drive Suite 200, The Colony, TX 75056, USA
* Corresponding author.
E-mail address: snodgrass@hypospadias.com

Urol Clin N Am 50 (2023) 447–453
https://doi.org/10.1016/j.ucl.2023.04.005

to specialists noted that over half had obstructive voiding or urine spraying.[6] We reported that 80% of men with uncorrected distal hypospadias had urine spraying. A third had lateral or ventral penile curvature that interfered with sexual intercourse, whereas one of every five with straight erections experienced pain during sex. Furthermore, 60% were bothered by the abnormal appearance of their penis.[7]

It is important to know the consequences, if any, of uncorrected, or unsuccessfully corrected, hypospadias when boys grow into men. Pediatric urologists advising families of newborns with distal hypospadias need this information to accurately counsel parents. They also need to know if reoperations should be done when initial repairs do not achieve a normal meatus or make the penis straight. Similarly, adult urologists should know if men presenting with hypospadias eventually accommodate to their situation or benefit from referral to surgeons experienced with adult hypospadias repair. Finally, with increasing scrutiny of genital surgery in children by activists and policy makers worldwide, a better understanding of the adult outcomes when boys are not repaired is essential.

WHAT DEFINES NORMAL VERSUS ABNORMAL ANATOMY?

As the goal of hypospadias surgery is to change abnormal into normal anatomy, it is important for urologists to know how to objectively make this distinction. Hutton and Babu[8] analyzed normal boys and reported glans fusion from the ventral lip of the meatus to the corona averaged 4.7 mm with a minimum of 2.5 mm. We have noted that glans fusion in adults averages 10 mm. Examples of normal glans fusion are shown in **Fig. 1**.

If little or no glans fusion correlates with abnormal function, then measuring glans fusion becomes an objective means to determine whether a boy with hypospadias should undergo repair, and if that correction should bring the neomeatus to a normal position. Similarly, this knowledge would advise if glans dehiscence should be corrected.

Urine Spraying

None of the 51 men with uncorrected hypospadias we evaluated had glans fusion, as seen in representative photos in **Fig. 2**, and 80% of them reported urine spraying (**Fig. 3**). Similarly, we found urine spraying in 60% of 82 men presenting with problems after childhood repair, which increased to 91% if they had no glans fusion.[9]

The glans normally encloses the meatus, serving as a nozzle on a hose to focus the stream. Accordingly, boys and men with normal anatomy do not spray, and neither do those who have normal glans fusion after hypospadias repair.

Spraying in infants or boys still in diapers is almost never reported by their parents. After toilet training spraying may initially be misinterpreted by them as inattentiveness or lack of aim. We have noticed that difficulties with the stream are first reported in boys with abnormal anatomy around age eight and are routine in teens and adults. Typically, they describe their stream as more compact when it is most forceful, but it sprays and splatters toward the end of urination as bladder pressures decrease or when they try to void with a partially filled bladder.

Urologists should not minimize the impact of an abnormal stream. Many patients described ongoing concern that their stream would soil their pants, or the shoes of someone standing at an adjacent urinal, even if these occurred infrequently, because it was unpredictable. Some first checked if a public toilet was empty before standing at a urinal and used a stall when it was occupied. Others pressed abnormally close to the urinal to keep the stream inside it. One man urinated into his hand to direct the stream so that he could stand to void. Given that men normally void six to eight times a day, it is not surprising that frustration with the basic act of urination was the chief complaint in our series. Many summarized their motivation to see a urologist as "just wanting to pee right."

Their experience also makes clear that simply asking if a man urinates standing may not capture the true nature of his voiding. Repair that achieves normal glans fusion stops urine spraying and splattering.

Sexual Dysfunction

Sexual dysfunction arises from penile curvature and/or from other anatomic differences, including exposed urethral mucosa from the abnormally enlarged meatus or a scrotal web extending up the penile shaft.

In our series of men with uncorrected distal hypospadias, one of every three had penile curvature that averaged 36° (15–65). This was mostly ventral with two patients having lateral bending. This curvature made penetration difficult for one patient and caused discomfort to the sexual partner in another five. Most reported that they avoided various sexual positions because of the bending.

Some men without penile curvature also complained of pain during sexual activity. One of every four with straight erections had irritation of the exposed urethral mucosa, which Leunback and

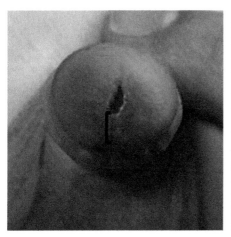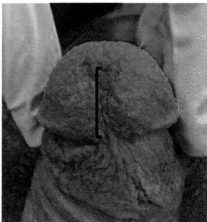

Fig. 1. Normal glans fusion in a boy and a man. The brackets indicate the distance from the lower lip of the meatus to the corona.

colleagues[6] noted was especially likely in those with megameatus intact prepuce (MIP) hypospadias. Another two men in our study had scrotal webs extending up the penile shaft that chafed their wives, whereas one other man had pain from a tight foreskin.

The prevalence of penile curvature in distal hypospadias is not well-defined. We previously reported ventral and lateral curvature occurred in 11% and 2% of distal hypospadias patients, respectively, and that all ventral bending was less than 30°.[10] However, this tally excluded boys with a distal meatus and bending thought to exceed 30°, who were classified as proximal hypospadias variants. In addition, we did not objectively measure curvature at that time. Consequently, we underestimated both the likelihood a boy with a distal meatus has penile curvature and the severity of that curvature, when present.

Our finding that a third of men with uncorrected distal hypospadias had penile curvature is telling. None reported surgical correction was postponed until adulthood because of curvature—rather, their birth defect was not considered a future risk warranting repair. A recent study similarly reported ventral curvature in 31% of distal hypospadias.[11]

The curvature we found averaged 36° with a range measured by goniometry from 15° to 65°. The functional importance of his bending was emphasized by a report that curvature of only 20° caused difficulties with sexual intercourse, and more unhealthy mental days, than men who had a straight penis experienced.[12] Similarly, a study of adults with congenital curvature which used a protractor to measure bending reported that 25° prompted men to request surgical straightening.[13]

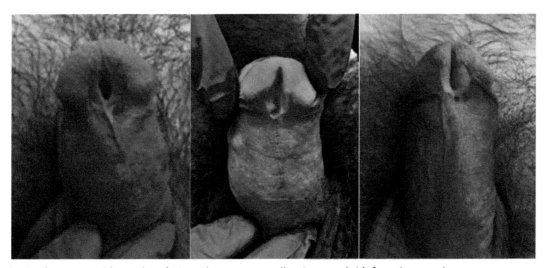

Fig. 2. Three men with no glans fusion. These men are all at increased risk for urine spraying.

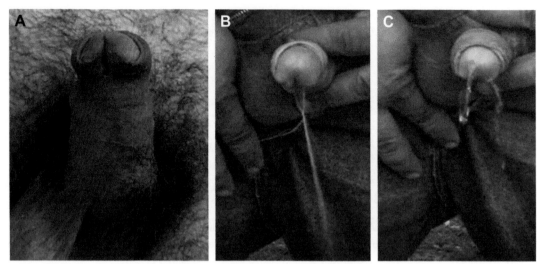

Fig. 3. Deflected and splattering stream. (*A*) Meatus with no glans fusion. (*B*) Initial stream is deflected down and spreads into a fan shape. (*C*) Near the end of voiding, the stream splatters.

Penile Appearance

None of the men in our series with uncorrected hypospadias gave a chief complaint of abnormal appearance of their penis. However, despite an average age of 42 years (18–63) and with many of them married or in a stable relationship, 61% said their different appearance was another motivation to consider surgery. Several admitted that they delayed intimacy and had fewer sexual partners specifically from concern that a new lover would ask what was wrong with their penis.

Men presenting with complications related to their childhood hypospadias repair also commonly complain of their abnormal appearance. Their concerns relate to a subglanular meatus, glans scars from epithelial stitching, or abnormalities of the penile shaft skin such as uneven circumcision scars, cross-hatched scars, suture sinuses, bumps, and hair on the shaft from scrotal flaps.

ARE SYMPTOMATIC MEN REPRESENTATIVE OR OUTLIERS?

Before conclusions can be drawn, the question of whether men presenting with these concerns are representative or outliers of men with uncorrected hypospadias has to be addressed.

This is especially important regarding urine spraying, as this was the chief complaint causing them to seek attention. Men do not normally spray, and if the glans serves to focus the stream, it stands to reason that those whose meatus is not enclosed by the glans would have an increased risk for spraying. None of our patients had glans

fusion, and most of them complained they could not reliably aim their stream. The fact this was also observed in 91% of men with complications after childhood repair who had little or no glans fusion further supports that conclusion.

Ching and colleagues[5] similarly reported most of the men with uncorrected hypospadias in their smaller series had urinary complaints which included spraying. Even Dodds and colleagues,[3] who wrote that men become accustomed to their hypospadias over time, admitted that a third of their patients described urine spraying.

Nevertheless, some still wonder if the men we evaluated were somehow different than others with uncorrected hypospadias because they presented to a specialty center wanting surgery. However, a third of those 51 men did not have surgery; some never scheduling repair after their consultation and others canceling it without explanation. There were no differences in men who underwent repair and these who did not regarding their mean age (42 vs 37 years), urine spraying (82% vs 80%), ventral curvature (30% vs 33%; mean 33°vs 34°), sexual dysfunction (33% vs 53%), or concerns for penile appearance (60% vs 63%).[7]

Even if there are other men with uncorrected hypospadias who do not have urinary or sexual dysfunction and are not bothered by their appearance, our findings, and those of others we cite above, undeniably indicate that distal hypospadias causes significant functional penile problems in at least some males born with it. This possibility must be disclosed to parents as part of informed consent, even if the surgeon believes distal hypospadias is little more than "cosmetic."

WHO BENEFITS FROM A DISTAL REPAIR?

If the goal of hypospadias surgery is to make abnormal anatomy normal, then measurement of glans fusion is important to determine who needs surgery and when repair is successful. A boy with a glanular meatus with normal glans fusion does not need a hypospadias urethroplasty (**Fig. 4**), whereas one with subnormal or no glans fusion can be recommended for repair because of the risk for urine spraying.

Similarly, the possibility that as many as a third of boys with distal hypospadias have ventral curvature, and reports that 20° is sufficient to cause sexual dysfunction and worry about their penis, mandates the urologist rule out curvature before concluding there is no functional reason to recommend repair.

IS A CORONAL MEATUS SUFFICIENT FOR PROXIMAL HYPOSPADIAS REPAIR?

Recent reports from Texas Children's, Boston Children's, and children's hospital of philadelphia (CHOP)[14–16] finding complications in 50% or more of patients after proximal repairs have led some surgeons to conclude the standard of making a normal penis is too high in these patients. Rather, they convert proximal into distal hypospadias, intentionally leaving the meatus on the corona or lower. However, this leaves the neomeatus without any glans fusion and therefore creates risk the patient will have urine spraying. A nonterminal meatus also increases the likelihood that

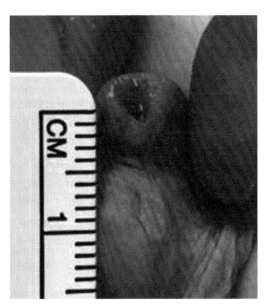

Fig. 4. Glanular hypospadias with normal glans fusion. Because he has normal anatomy, distal urethroplasty is not necessary.

the boy grown into a teen and adult will be dissatisfied with the different appearance of his penis.

The patients in these series underwent one- and two-stage flap repairs. Years ago WS also had a high complication rate using these same methods, which prompted a change to staged graft urethroplasties. We reported consecutive proximal repairs to a normal glanular meatus by staged grafts had complications in 23%. Those were fistulas and glans dehiscence, and overall success increased to 98% once those were repaired.[17]

Others using staged graft repairs also published up to 50% fewer complications than reported using flaps.[18–20] Knowledge that repairing to a nonterminal meatus will result in future spraying in at least some, if not most, these boys emphasize the need to create a normally positioned neomeatus, even if that requires a change from flap to graft techniques.

DO CHILDHOOD REPAIRS DETERIORATE DURING PUBERTY?

Recently, concern has arisen that a successful childhood hypospadias repair might develop complications, especially ventral curvature or fistulas, during puberty and require reoperation.[21,22] This has led some parents to question repairing hypospadias before growth is complete.

To evaluate this possibility, we reviewed consecutive teens and adults with complications after childhood repair to determine when those occurred. We found that 80% developed before puberty, with only 5% occurring pubertal growth, two fistulas and two strictures. The remaining 15% presented with new obstructive symptoms from meatal stenosis or urethral stricture at a mean age of 47 years,[8] which was similar to Barbagli's report that strictures can develop years after surgery.[23]

We have yet to encounter a patient who developed new or recurrent penile curvature during puberty. To our knowledge, there is only one published mention of this occurrence and that came from a center that used chordee excision for penile straightening and did not perform artificial erection afterward to determine its efficacy. We have seen many teens with ventral curvature after childhood repair who stated it was present long before puberty but was dismissed or overlooked by their urologist until their penile growth made the situation undeniable.

ARE HYPOSPADIAS REPAIRS IN ADULTS SUCCESSFUL?

It is commonly believed that complications increase when repairs are done in older patients. However, we studied outcomes in 669 consecutive prepubertal boys ages 3 months to 12 years using logistic regression, which determined meatal location and reoperation—but not age—correlated with complications.[24]

We then performed the first study directly comparing outcomes between cohorts of boys and men undergoing primary and reoperative hypospadias repair.[25] This was done to address concerns that risks for complications were greater in adults, leading many adult reconstructive urologists to end the urethroplasty near the corona. We found no difference in outcomes in adults versus children for either primary or reoperative repair, which also counters the advice of many general urologists to men presenting with hypospadias that they should learn to live with their situation because the likelihood for poor outcomes is too high.

Most of the men presenting with uncorrected hypospadias have a distal meatus, and others have also reported successful TIP repair in them.[2–6,8–13,26–28]

Therefore, general urologists encountering men with uncorrected hypospadias should not discourage them from surgery, and reconstructive urologists who choose to do these operations should have the goal of making the penis normal.

WHAT HAPPENS WHEN REPAIR IS POSTPONED UNTIL ADULTHOOD?

If outcomes from adult repairs are equivalent to those in children, activists and policy makers question the need and ethics for earlier repair in patients who cannot give their own consent.

Although we have found surgical outcomes are the same regardless of age, anyone who has routinely managed teens and adults with uncorrected or unsuccessfully corrected hypospadias has seen how the entire experience is different. Despite their desire to have a normal penis, older patients arrive to preoperative consultations and on the day of surgery very anxious and often hypertensive. Before then they have worried how to explain their upcoming absence to coworkers and supervisors, not wanting to mention surgery on their penis. Men also hurt more after surgery, particularly suffering from painful nocturnal erections which cannot be prevented. We have also noticed that, as a group, they are not patient with their recovery and often become frustrated when they have not returned to normal within a few weeks. In addition, many intensively study their penis and worry about normal postoperative swelling, small skin bumps, erythema of the skin incision, and so forth. Men also commonly complain that surgery has made their penis shorter. So many who have had prior surgery manifest PTSD-type reactions that we strongly encourage preoperative counseling.

Although we and others have reported that foreskin reconstruction can be done in nearly all boys with distal hypospadias, that is, not true in adults. The foreskin grows comparatively less during puberty, often leaving insufficient skin to reconstruct if a man wants a normal uncircumcised appearance.

Surgery is also more difficult in men because of the increased size of the penis and its blood vessels, which means that they bleed more. Men additionally have increased risk for postoperative bleeding creating scrotal hematomas, which we encountered in half our patients until we imposed strict bed rest during their first 12 to 18 hours after surgery.

Men undergoing reoperations that include oral graft harvest suffer more than boys having the same procedure—the pain in their mouths typically greater than in their penis.

Furthermore, we have never had a teen or adult say he was pleased that his surgery was postponed so that he could make the decision for it. Rather, many are angry after learning their birth defect could have been corrected when they were young and would have no recollection of it. By delaying surgery, they had to cope with the realization that their penis was not normal with no one available they wanted to discuss their concerns with. They did not want to talk to their friends, and certainly not their parents, about their penis. So they worried in isolation. In addition, many adults admit they avoided relationships when they were younger that might lead to intimacy for fear what a lover would think about their penis. Through all this many, even most, have had to deal day after day with an unpredictable urine stream that might spray during any void.

Considering all these factors, it would be a rare situation when postponing repair until adulthood is an advantage.

SUMMARY

These data and observations reinforce several conclusions regarding hypospadias and its repair.

1. Birth defects of the penis are best corrected in childhood.
2. The goal of surgery is to make the abnormal anatomy normal to best ensure normal urinary and sexual function.
3. Normal esthetics are also important to patients born with hypospadias, meaning surgeons should avoid incisions outside the median raphe and circumcision lines, use only penile skin to

cover the penis, and avoid glanular epithelial stitches which can leave scars and divots.

4. Successful repair making the penis straight with a normal neomeatus and symmetric circumferential coverage with penile skin has little risk for future complications.

5. Adults who present with uncorrected hypospadias, or complications after prior repairs, can still have successful surgery that includes making a normal neomeatus.

These lessons that adult patients teach urologists about hypospadias can be summarized by the conclusion that boys born with this birth defect want to grow into men with a normal penis.

DISCLOSURE

The authors have no disclosures.

REFERENCES

1. Snodgrass W, Bush N. TIP hypospadias repair: a pediatric urology indicator operation. J Ped Urol 2016;12:11–8.

2. Fichtner J, Filipas D, Mottrie AM, et al. Analysis of meatal location in 500 men: wide variation questions need for meatal advancement in all pediatric anterior hypospadias cases. J Urol 1995;154:833–4.

3. Dodds PR, Batter SJ, Shield DE, et al. Adaptation of adults to uncorrected hypospadias. Urology 2008; 71:682–5.

4. Schlomer B, Breyer B, Copp H, et al. Do adult men with untreated hypospadias have adverse outcomes? A pilot study using a social media advertised survey. J Pediatr Urol 2014;10:672–9.

5. Ching CB, Wood HM, Ross JH, et al. The Cleveland Clinic experience with adult hypospadias patients undergoing repair: their presentation and a new classification system. BJU Int 2010;107:1142–6.

6. Leunback TL, Skott M, Ernst A, et al. Referral patterns, clinical features and management of uncorrected hypospadias in a series of adult men. J Pediatr Urol 2022;18(4):480.e1–7.

7. Bush N and Snodgrass W: Does uncorrected distal hypospadias cause problems in adults? submitted 2023.

8. Hutton KAR, Babu R. Normal anatomy of the external urethral meatus in boys: implications for hypospadias repair. BJU Int 2007;100:161–3.

9. Snodgrass W, Bush N. Do new complications develop during puberty after childhood hypospadias repair? J Urol 2022;208:696–701.

10. Snodgrass W, Bush N. Hypospadias. In: Wein A, editor. Campbell's urology. 10th Edition; 2011.

11. Stojanovic B, Bizic M, Majstorovic M, et al. Penile curvature incidence in hypospadias: can it be determined? Adv Urol 2011;2011:813205.

12. Menon V, Breyer B, Copp HL, et al. Do adult men with untreated ventral penile curvature have adverse outcomes? J Pediatr Urol 2016;12:31.e1-7.

13. Greenfield JM, Lucas S, Levine LA. Factors affecting the loss of length associated with tunica albuginea plication for correction of penile curvature. J Urol 2006;175:238–41.

14. Stanasel I, Le HK, Bilgutay A, et al. Complications following staged hypospadias repair using transposed prepucial skin flaps. J Urol 2015;194:512–6.

15. McNamara ER, Schaeffer AJ, Logvinenko T, et al. Management of proximal hypospadias with 2-stage repair: 20-year experience. J Urol 2015;194:1080–5.

16. Long CJ, Chu DI, Tenny RW, et al. Intermediate-term followup of proximal hypospadias repair reveals high complication rate. J Urol 2017;197:852–8.

17. Snodgrass W, Bush N. Staged tubularized autograft repair for primary proximal hypospadias with 30-degree of greater ventral curvature. J Urol 2017;198: 680–6.

18. Ferro F, Zaccara A, Spagnoli A, et al. Skin graft for 2-stage treatment of severe hypospadias: back to the future? J Urol 2002;168:1730–3.

19. Castagnetti M, Zhapa E, Rigamonti W. Primary severe hypospadias: comparison of reoperative rates and parental perception urinary symptoms and cosmetic outcomes among 4 repairs. J Urol 2013; 189:1508–13.

20. Pippi Salle JL, Sayed S, Salle A, et al. Proximal hypospadias: a persistent challenge. Single institution outcome analysis of three surgical techniques over a 10-year period. J Pediatr Urol 2016;12:28 e1–e7.

21. Ekmark AN, Svensson H, Arnbjornsson E, et al. Postpubertal examination after hypospadias repair is necessary to evaluate the success of primary reconstruction. Eur J Pediar Surg 2013;23:304–11.

22. Johnston A, Jibara GA, Purves JT, et al. Delayed presentation of urethrocutaneous fistula after hypospadias repair. J Pediatr Surg 2020;55:2206–8.

23. Barbagli G, De Angelis M, Palminteri E, et al. Failed hypospadias repair presenting in adults. Eur Urol 2006;49:887–95.

24. Bush N, Holzer M, Zhang S, Snodgrass W. Age does not impact risk for urethroplasty complications after tubularized incised plate repair of hypospadias in prepubertal boys. J Pediatr Urol 2013;9:252–6.

25. Snodgrass W, Villanueva C, Bush N. Primary and reoperative hypospadias repair in adults–are results different than in children? J Urol 2014;192:1730–3.

26. Sharma G. Tubularized-incised plate urethroplasty in adults. BJU Int 2005;95:374–6.

27. Sahin C, Yesildal C. Adult distal hypospadias repair is safe and easy. Andrologia 2022;54:e14398.

28. Bush N, Snodgrass W. Does uncorrected distal hypospadias cause problems in adults? submitted to. Dove Press; 2023.

Wilms Tumor

Amanda F. Saltzman, MD[a], Nicholas G. Cost, MD[b,c],*,
Rodrigo L.P. Romao, MD[d,e]

KEYWORDS

• Wilms tumor • Nephroblastoma • Renal tumor • Nephrectomy • Urologic oncology

KEY POINTS

• Wilms tumor is the most common malignant renal tumor in childhood.
• The most important prognostic feature in Wilms tumor is histology (favorable histology vs anaplasia).
• Multimodal therapy for Wilms tumor is associated with a good prognosis that allows for a current focus on risk-adapted therapy to allow for maximizing oncology outcomes while minimizing therapeutic morbidity.

INTRODUCTION

Wilms tumor (WT), or nephroblastoma, is the most common primary malignant renal tumor of childhood. It is an embryonal tumor that develops from remnants of immature kidney. There are approximately 500 new WT cases diagnosed in the United States every year.[1] Advances in multimodal therapy including surgery, chemotherapy, and radiation therapy given according to risk stratification have allowed most patients to achieve survival rates in excess of 90%.[2] The focus of the most recently completed cooperative group clinical trials was on reducing the morbidity of treatment of low-risk patients, reserving more intensive treatment of high-risk patients (ie, anaplastic Wilms, loss of heterozygosity (LOH) at chromosome 1p and 16q, post-chemotherapy blastemal predominant histology) for whom survival remains poor.[2] In general, future trials will continue to pursue improving oncological outcomes as well as minimizing treatment-related toxicity when feasible.

PRESENTATION

Most children with sporadic WT present with a palpable abdominal mass that is first noticed by a caregiver or primary care physician. Patients are often otherwise healthy, which is helpful in establishing a differential diagnosis with neuroblastoma. Other symptoms such as hypertension, hematuria, and flank pain can be observed in 20% to 25% of cases.[3] Presentation after blunt abdominal trauma with abdominal/flank pain and blood loss has been observed anecdotally, but its incidence has never been formally studied.

Patients with WT usually present at 3 to -5 years old and most cases are diagnosed before age less than 10 years. African American children seem to be at higher risk of developing WT, and patients of Asian descent have the lowest risk of WT. Although there are several well-described syndromes associated with an increased chance of developing WT, this is seen in the minority of patients with WT. The WT1 gene is critically involved with the development of WT. This is found on the short arm of chromosome 11 (11p13). WT1 is a tumor suppressor gene that codes for a transcription factor that is linked to embryologic genitourinary development. Homozygous mutations of WT1, or nearby coding regions, very often results in the patient developing WT.[4,5]

Multiple genetic syndromes may predispose children to WT, as listed in **Table 1**. Patients with

[a] Department of Urology, University of Kentucky, Lexington, KY, USA; [b] Division of Urology, Department of Surgery, University of Colorado School of Medicine, 13123 East 16th Avenue, B 463, Aurora, CO 80045, USA; [c] Surgical Oncology Program, Children's Hospital Colorado, 13123 East 16th Avenue, B 463, Aurora, CO 80045, USA; [d] Department of Surgery, IWK Health Centre, Dalhousie University, Halifax, Canada; [e] Department of Urology, IWK Health Centre, Dalhousie University, Halifax, Canada
* Corresponding author.
E-mail address: nicholas.cost@childrenscolorado.org

Urol Clin N Am 50 (2023) 455–464
https://doi.org/10.1016/j.ucl.2023.04.008

Table 1
Wilms tumor predisposition syndromes

Syndrome	Genetics	Associated Features	Risk of WT (%)
Wilms tumor Aniridia Gu Anomalies syndrom (WAGR)	11p13 *WT1, PAX13*	WT Aniridia Genital abnormalities Mental delay	98
Denys–Drash	*WT1*	WT Genital abnormalities Renal failure/nephropathy (mesangial sclerosis)	74

Beckwith–Wiedemann	11p15.5 *WT2*	Prenatal and postnatal
		  overgrowth
		Hemihypertrophy
		  (growth asymmetry)
		Macroglossia
		Anterior abdominal
		  wall defects (omphalocele)
		Ear creases/pits
			7

Frasier syndrome	*WT1*	WT
		Nephropathy focal
		  segmental glomerular
		  sclerosis (FSGS)
		Genital abnormalities
		Gonadoblastoma/Germ cell
		  neoplasia in situ (GCNIS)
			6

predisposition syndromes and bilateral tumors typically present at earlier ages than those without. Screening protocols are often used for these patients to attempt to diagnose tumors at an earlier stage, but whether these impacts overall outcomes is unclear. In general, screening protocols involve an abdominal ultrasound every 3 to 6 months until age 7 to 10 years.[6]

DIAGNOSTIC WORKUP

Workup begins with a complete history and physical examination. Careful questioning regarding signs of predisposition syndromes, end stage renal disease (ESRD), and family history is important. Determining if hematuria is or is not present may affect surgical planning. Physical examination is critical, looking for signs of hemihypertrophy, genital malformations, and eye anomalies.

Laboratory workup should include a complete blood count, comprehensive metabolic panel including liver function tests, urinalysis, and coagulation tests. A small subset (2%–4%) of patients with WT may have an acquired von Willebrand's disease, which is useful to know preoperatively.[7]

The goals of preoperative imaging include staging and preoperative planning. From a staging perspective, it is important to look for free fluid, which may be a sign of rupture. The presence of ureteral or inferior vena cava (IVC) tumor thrombus is also important. It is also important to assess the contralateral kidney, as bilateral masses prompt preoperative chemotherapy rather than a direct trip to the operating room.

When a patient presents with a palpable mass, imaging should begin with a renal ultrasound (US). The differential for an upper quadrant mass is wide and includes kidney, liver, and adrenal tumors, along with a host of other benign conditions. Beginning with a readily available, low-cost, low-risk imaging study will allow tailoring of subsequent imaging to minimize the chance that extraneous studies will be ordered, which may result in increased radiation exposure.[1] Staging requires a computed tomography (CT) of the chest to assess for metastatic disease. The abdomen and pelvis need to be imaged as well, either through CT or MRI with intravenous (IV) contrast in a single phase (**Fig. 1**). MRI is preferred for bilateral tumors due to the increased need for surveillance and desire to minimize radiation exposure. Findings to note include tumor thrombus, ureteral thrombus, enlarged lymph node (LNs) and if there are any anomalies of the contralateral kidney. Although imaging findings suspicious for preoperative rupture and lymphadenopathy have low

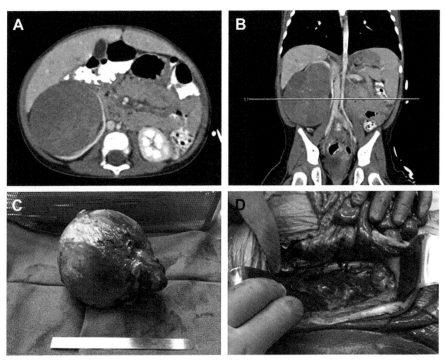

Fig. 1. (*A*) Axial and (*B*) coronal view of CT scan showing a right-sided Wilms tumor with images of the specimen (*C*), and resection bed of right retroperitoneum (*D*).

sensitivity (CT 76% and MRI 53%) and are not used for final staging, it can provide guidance what the surgeon may encounter in the operating room.[8] The assessment of the involvement of other organs is also important, but keep in mind that WT usually displaces surrounding structures, rarely invades them.

INITIAL MANAGEMENT

Management of a renal mass suspicious for WT generally centers on surgery. Generally, upfront open radical nephrectomy is the standard treatment, but there are several situations in which neoadjuvant chemotherapy should be considered and/or pursued. Although WT usually push surrounding structures away, they rarely invade them. If, in the surgeon's opinion, there is concern for invasion into surrounding structures or the tumor is not resectable, or it is unsafe to put the patient under anesthesia (eg, massive pulmonary metastases), neoadjuvant chemotherapy can be used to shrink the tumor to avoid resection of surrounding organs. Similarly, if there is an IVC thrombus above the hepatic veins, neoadjuvant chemotherapy can be used to shrink the thrombus to allow future resection without the use of cardiac bypass.[9]

Patients with bilateral tumors, known predisposition syndromes or a solitary kidney, should undergo neoadjuvant chemotherapy, without biopsy, to try to make the tumors more amenable to nephron-sparing surgery (NSS).[10] The major long-term issue that these patients face is ESRD, so it is imperative to minimize the amount of kidney excised and this is achieved using neoadjuvant chemotherapy. Generally, patients are given a regimen of vincristine, actinomycin-d with or without doxorubicin for 6 weeks (two cycles), and then imaging is repeated. Currently, the response and potential resectability are assessed. A partial response is defined by at least a 30% decrease in longest axial dimension. If there has been a response and NSS is feasible, surgical can be pursued. If there has been a partial response but NSS is not feasible, an additional 6 weeks of neoadjuvant chemotherapy should be recommended. If there has not been at least a partial response, consideration for tissue diagnosis via biopsy should be recommended to assess for either anaplasia or non-WT pathology. This can be done by percutaneous or open approaches with open having an improved likelihood of identifying anaplasia.

There are a few situations that urologists need to be aware of. Although the typical WT patient is 2 to 5 years of age, patients outside this age range may harbor different pathology. A renal mass in a patient less than 6 months of age is likely a congenital mesoblastic nephroma (CMN). CMN is generally benign; however, management is early radical nephrectomy with LN sampling, such as WT. Conversely, a renal mass in a patient greater than 10 years of age is more likely to be renal cell carcinoma (RCC).[4] Treatment still centers on surgery, but the discussion of preoperative biopsy, minimally invasive techniques, and NSS may be considered.

Staging is finalized using several factors, namely dictated by the pathologist and surgeon. Surgeon findings are emphasized over imaging due to poor sensitivity of cross-sectional imaging to estimate things such as spillage, lymphadenopathy, surrounding tissue invasion, and so forth.

All specimens including kidney, LNs, and other tissue must be sent for histologic assessment fresh, not in formalin. Exposure to formalin will limit the tests that can be done as some tests require fresh tissue. If the tissue is being sent "after hours," the surgeon should preoperatively coordinate with the pathology as to how the specimens will be sent to allow all appropriate tests to be conducted.

OPERATIVE MANAGEMENT
Radical Nephrectomy

This should be done transperitoneal through a large horizontal abdominal incision that usually crosses the midline. A horizontal incision is used because young children are generally wider than they are long, so it is difficult to reach the lateral extent of the abdomen through a standard midline incision. Avoiding the flank approach decreases the chance of intraoperative spill due to inadequate exposure.

On opening the abdomen, peritoneal fluid should be assessed. Bloody fluid is highly suspicious for preoperative rupture. Next, the peritoneal surfaces should be palpated, along with the liver, for any nodules suspicious for tumor implants. If palpated, these should be excised and sent for pathology. These sites should be marked with metal clips to watch these areas during surveillance. The routine exploration of the contralateral kidney is unnecessary as imaging should provide adequate assessment.

The colon is then mobilized medially to expose the retroperitoneum. Early ligation of the hilum should not be pursued if technically difficult or dangerous due to tumor size or extensive LN involvement. The ureter is identified and ligated as distally as possible, using a dissolvable stitch. The ureter is then traced proximally to the renal hilum. The surgeon should note any suspicious lymphadenopathy. The lateral and superior attachments of the kidney are then released keeping Gerota's fascia intact. The adrenal gland may be left in place if it is not abutting the tumor. If there is concern of adrenal involvement preoperatively or intraoperatively, the adrenal should be resected en bloc to avid spillage. It is very important to handle the kidney/tumor with care to avoid intraoperative spill, as this upstages the patient and mandates therapeutic intensification. The renal vein and artery are identified and the renal vein should be palpated for a thrombus. The vessels are then ligated. The kidney is freed and should be passed off the field en bloc without disruption. The tumor capsule should be examined by the surgeon and any disruptions noted as suspicious for rupture.

If there is concern that gross tumor remains, it is helpful for the surgeon to mark these areas with metal clips to potentially guide radiation therapy and to mark areas to watch on surveillance. These clips can interfere with subsequent imaging, so they should be limited to what is necessary.

Lymph Node Sampling

Next, LNs need to be sampled. This is a critical, and too often omitted, portion of the surgical treatment of WT. Regional LNs should be sampled, but a formal LN dissection is not necessary. LNs should be sampled from the para-aortic space on the left and the paracaval space on the right. Tumors of both sides should also have interaortocaval LNs sampled as there is cross-over spread.[11] As far as how many LNs need to be sampled, this is less clear, but current data suggested somewhere between 6 and 10 LNs should be the goal.[12,13]

Partial Nephrectomy/Nephron-Sparing Surgery

This begins similar to a radical nephrectomy as far as approach, incision and initial steps. The incision may need to be slightly longer given that both sides may need to be accessed. Importantly, it is ok to perform bilateral NSS in the same setting.

Partial nephrectomy involves control of the hilum in case conversion to radical nephrectomy will be needed. Gerota's fascia is opened, unlike a radical nephrectomy, and overlying fat is removed. Intraoperative US can be used to help localize the tumor, and recent studies have found that indocyanine green (ICG) may be helpful as well. Tumors are resected with a goal of achieving grossly negative margins but also leaving as much renal tissue as possible. After removal of the tumor any bleeding vessels can be suture ligated with *absorbable* suture. If there is transection of the collecting system, a watertight closure with fine absorbable suture is recommended. Intraoperative consideration should be given to placing a ureteral stent and retroperitoneal drain if there is concern for a resulting postoperative urine leak. Renorraphy can be done by bringing the parenchyma back over the defect anchoring the sutures in the renal capsule.

Although control of the renal vessels is recommended, in young children, the renal vessels are very small and delicate. Care should be taken to not place too much traction on the vessels as this can raise intimal flaps and impair renal blood flow. It is also important to consider using hand clamping rather than hilar clamping (artery with or without vein), as there is a high risk of thrombosis of the small vessels. The use of cold ischemia is rare as it has significant thermal effects on small children.

LN sampling should be performed, using the same method as above. This is critical for staging and guiding subsequent therapy.

Minimally Invasive Surgery

Per childrens oncology group (COG) guidelines, this is generally avoided. In practice, most of these tumors will present as large palpable masses that are not amenable to NSS. The use of minimally invasive surgery (MIS) in WT has been associated with an increased risk of rupture and an increased chance that LN sampling will be omitted.

In contrast, the international society of pediatric oncology (SIOP) UMBRELLA protocol has a very narrow cohort of patients where MIS can be used. These patients have peripheral tumors that do not cross the midline. Importantly, all patients are treated with neoadjuvant chemotherapy, so it is presumed that their tumors are smaller than if resected immediately.

Biopsy

Per COG guidelines, biopsy is considered a local spill and will upstage the patient to stage III given the increased risk of local recurrence seen with tumor rupture/spill. This then mandates radiation and doxorubicin, which are both associated with more late effects. However, data to support that biopsy is associated with increased rates of local recurrence are poor using modern renal biopsy techniques.

Despite the probable safety of biopsy, a group from the United Kingdom examined the use of biopsy to determine which patients should undergo upfront surgery versus neoadjuvant chemotherapy (per SIOP protocols). They found that biopsy changed initial management in less than 5% of cases and have abandoned this practice, favoring neoadjuvant chemotherapy as initial treatment.[14] Although biopsy is likely safe, it is unlikely to change management and it still mandates therapeutic intensification using COG protocols.

Vascular Tumor Thrombus

Renal vein or IVC thrombus will likely be seen on preoperative imaging, which will allow the urologist to prepare for this. The renal vein should always be palpated before ligation to verify there is no thrombus and to allow resection without spillage. In case of uncertainty, intraoperative ultrasound can be used to evaluate the renal vein and IVC (**Fig. 2**). Control of the renal vein and cava above and below the tumor with vessel loops or umbilical tape is helpful. The tumor and kidney

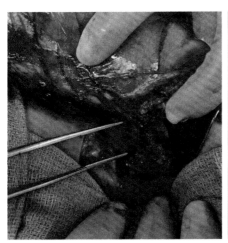 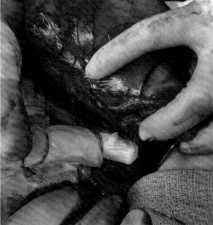

Fig. 2. Intraoperative image of a completely mobilized Wilms tumor with an intraoperative ultrasound being done of the renal vein to assess for any signs of venous tumor thrombus.

should be completely mobilized and the arterial supply taken before removing the thrombus. A venotomy is then made and the tumor pulled out of the vein. The tumor thrombus should not be transected if it can be avoided. In some instances, the tumor may be fixed to the vascular lumen and extraction is more difficult, so a larger venotomy may be required. A similar technique used for removing plaque for a carotid endarterectomy is helpful to lift the tumor off the vein wall using a Penfield elevator.

As mentioned above, consideration for neoadjuvant chemotherapy is indicated if the thrombus extends to or above retrohepatic vena cava.

Ureteral Tumor Thrombus

This is only detected on preoperative imaging in about 30% of cases that have ureteral tumor involvement but is present in 2% to 5% of patients. The urologist should be suspicious for a ureteral thrombus in patients with gross hematuria, hydronephrosis, urethral mass, or passage of tissue in the urine (**Fig. 3**). It may be worthwhile to consider cystoscopy and retrograde pyelogram to assess for this, or to assess for the extent of this thrombus so the ureteral occlusion can be distal to this level to allow resection without spillage.[15]

In cases of partial nephrectomy where the collecting system is expected to be entered, it may

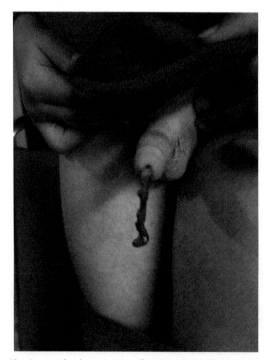

Fig. 3. Urethral extension of right-sided Wilms tumor.

be fruitful to begin with ureteral stent placement as the first part of the case.

Central Line Placement

In most cases, patients will receive adjuvant chemotherapy based on stage. It is often helpful to combine central line placement and nephrectomy. However, there are certain scenarios where patients may not need adjuvant chemotherapy, specifically the very low-risk group. These are patients age less than 2 years with favorable histology, stage I disease and tumor weighing less than 550 g. In the next COG studies, the criteria for omission of adjuvant chemotherapy will likely be widened, including more patients in this group.

In addition, very young patients are more likely to have benign tumors, and older patients are more likely to have RCC, neither of which require chemotherapy. In these cases, deferring central line placement may be appropriate. The use of intraoperative frozen section may help guide placement in these situations.

IMPORTANT DETAILS TO INCLUDE IN THE OPERATIVE REPORT FOR A PATIENT WITH WILMS TUMOR

- Type of incision
- Evidence of preoperative tumor rupture
- Palpation of surface of organs and peritoneum
- Evidence of intraoperative tumor spill
- Palpation of renal vein
- Obvious lymphadenopathy
- Gross margin status
- Location of removed lymph nodes
- Status of surrounding organs
- Surgical stage

POSTSURGICAL MANAGEMENT

Most patients will require adjuvant chemotherapy based on staging and risk stratification. The latter is grounded on histology (favorable vs anaplastic) and biology (LOH 1p and 16q) in the last generation of studies and also the presence of 1q gain moving forward. The backbone of favorable histology Wilms tumor (FHWT) treatment is vincristine, actinomycin-d, and doxorubicin. Higher risk FH and anaplastic tumors get exposed to more intensive therapy. The most common regimens used in the treatment of WT based on the last COG protocols (AREN0532, 0533, and 0534) are outlined. It is important to note that a new generation of studies for patients with FHWT is about to be launched soon with modifications to the schema below.

- EE4A: vincristine, actinomycin-d

Table 2
Summary of results of recent COG trials pertaining to *favorable histology*, unilateral Wilms tumor based on risk stratification

Stage	Risk Stratification	Treatment (Protocol)	Outcomes 4-Year Survival
I	Very low-risk Wilms tumor = age < 2 years, tumor weight < 550g	Surgery only (AREN0532)[16]	EFS 89.7% (84.1–95.2%) OS 100%
I and II	Standard risk *NO* LOH 1p and 16q	Nephrectomy, LN sampling, and EE4A	EFS 94% OS 98%
I and II	Higher risk LOH 1p and 16q	Nephrectomy, LN sampling, and DD4A (AREN 0533)[17]	EFS 87.3% (75.1–99.5%) OS 100%
III	*NO* LOH 1p and 16q	Nephrectomy, LN sampling, abdominal XRT (10.8 Gy), and regimen DD-4A[18]	EFS 88% (85–91%) OS 97% (95–98%)
IV	NO LOH 1p and 16q *AND* rapid complete response of lung nodules by week 6 of treatment	Nephrectomy, LN sampling, abdominal XRT if surgical stage III, *no lung radiation*, and regimen DD-4A (AREN0533)[19]	EFS 79.5% (71.2–87.8%) OS 96.1% (92.1–100%)
	NO LOH 1p and 16q *AND* incomplete response of lung nodules by week 6 of treatment	Nephrectomy + LN sampling, abdominal XRT (10.8 Gy), lung XRT (12 Gy), and regimen M (AREN0533)[19]	EFS 88.5% (81.8–95.3%) OS 95.4% (90.9–99.8%)
III or IV	LOH 1p and 16q	Nephrectomy + LN sampling, abdominal XRT (10.8 Gy), lung XRT (12 Gy), and regimen M (AREN0533)[17]	EFS 90.2% (81.7–98.6%) OS 96.1% (90.5–100%)

- DD4A: vincristine, actinomycin-d, doxorubicin
- Regimen M: vincristine, actinomycin-d, doxorubicin, cyclophosphamide, etoposide
- Revised[a] regimen UH1: vincristine, doxorubicin, cyclophosphamide, carboplatin, and etoposide plus radiotherapy
- Revised[a] regimen UH2: UH1 including a vincristine/irinotecan window

Patients with FHWT and a stage III designation will receive radiotherapy. Treatment will be directed to the flank or whole abdomen, depending on the reasoning behind a stage III label. For example, patients who are stage III due to nodal involvement or positive margins will be exposed to flank irradiation; however, patients with preoperative tumor rupture will receive whole abdominal radiation.

OUTCOMES
Unilateral, Non-syndromic Wilms Tumor

Tables 2 and 3 summarize the most recently published outcomes from COG renal tumor committee (RTC) studies related to favorable histology and

anaplastic unilateral WT. The key highlights in this group of patients are summarized below.

- There is a very low risk group of young patients with small tumors who can be successfully treated with surgery alone, thus sparing them from the long-term effects of systemic treatment.
- Patients with FHWT and favorable biology (no LOH 1p and 16q) harboring metastatic disease to the lungs who have a complete response to chemotherapy by week 6 of treatment can be spared lung radiation. Those with an incomplete response have improved outcomes with intensified chemotherapy and lung radiation compared with historical controls.
- Patients with combined LOH of both 1p and 16q make up only 5% of the total patients with FHWT; nonetheless, they experience improved outcomes with intensified therapy compared with historical controls.

Table 3 summarizes the most recently published outcomes from COG RTC studies for patients with

---

[a]Doses were revised due to initial toxicity.

Table 3
Summary of results of recent COG trials pertaining to unilateral *anaplastic* Wilms tumor

Stage	Type of Anaplasia	Treatment (Protocol)	Outcomes 4-Year Survival
I	Focal or diffuse	Nephrectomy, LN sampling, flank XRT (10.8 Gy), and regimen DD4-A (AREN0321)[20]	EFS 100% OS 100%
II	Diffuse	Nephrectomy, LN sampling, flank XRT, and revised regimen UH1 (AREN0321)[21]	EFS 86.7% (68.8–100%) OS 86.2% (68–100%)
III	Diffuse	Nephrectomy, LN sampling, abdominal XRT (whole abdomen or flank), and revised regimen UH1 (AREN0321)[21]	EFS 80.9% (65.8–96%) OS 88.6% (76.4–100%)
IV	Diffuse	Nephrectomy, LN sampling, abdominal XRT (whole abdomen or flank), XRT to metastatic sites, and revised regimen UH2[21]	EFS 41.7% (29.6–90.4%) OS 49.2% (41.6–98.4%)

Notes: Bilateral WT, bilaterally predisposed WT (unilateral tumors in patients with predisposition syndromes or solitary kidney), and diffuse hyperplastic perilobar nephroblastomatosis (DHPLN).

evidence of focal or diffuse anaplastic WT (focal anaplasia [FA] or diffuse anaplasia [DA]).

Results of the first ever protocol dedicated to the treatment of bilateral, unilateral multicentric, or bilaterally predisposed unilateral WT have recently become available. In AREN0534, there were three arms pertaining to this group of patients.

Bilateral Wilms tumor

In the first arm, patients with synchronous lesions larger than 1 cm affecting both kidneys were treated with neoadjuvant three-drug (regimen vincristine, actinomycin-D, and doxorubicin) chemotherapy without a biopsy.[10] The feasibility of bilateral NSS was then assessed at 6 and 12 weeks. One of the objectives of the study was to make sure that surgical treatment was not delayed beyond 12 weeks of therapy initiation, a pattern that had been observed in previous cooperative trials.[22] This goal was achieved in 84% of participants and one-third of patients had surgery at 6 weeks post-chemotherapy initiation.

The 4-year survival for 189 patients with bilateral WT compared favorably with National Wilms tumor study 5 (NWTS5) (event free survival [EFS] 82% [73.5–90.8%], overall survival [OS] 94% [90.1–99.7%]). The only unmet target of AREN0534 was the rate of bilateral NSS, 39% vs the proposed 50%.[10] This area is subject of active research to predict feasibility and increase NSS rates in this particular group of patients at risk for long-term renal dysfunction.

Unilateral Wilms tumor in patients with multicentric tumors, predisposition syndromes, or solitary kidneys

This group was also treated with neoadjuvant chemotherapy (a two-drug regimen of vincristine and actinomycin-D) followed by NSS if feasible. Most of the patients had multicentric tumors (n = 10), Beckwith–Wiedemann syndrome (n = 9) or isolated hemihypertrophy (n = 9). EFS and OS for 34 patients were excellent at 94% (85%–100%) and 100%, respectively. Two patients experienced complete resolution of their tumors after chemotherapy. Out of the 32 who underwent surgery, only 12 had a complete nephrectomy.[23] This study corroborates the importance of looking for multicentric tumors and predisposition syndromes at the time of diagnosis.

Diffuse hyperplastic perilobar nephroblastomatosis

Diffuse hyperplastic perilobar nephroblastomatosis (DHPLN) represents a rare but significant issue affecting both kidneys. The condition has a typical appearance on cross-sectional imaging related to the presence of nephrogenic rests, which if left untreated will invariably progress to WT (**Fig. 4**). On the other hand, prolonged treatment with chemotherapy has been shown to lead to the development of anaplastic WT in some patients.

The AREN0534 enrolled patients with DHPLN in one of its arms and treated them with EE4A chemotherapy with close follow-up for selective surgery (preferably NSS if possible) if discrete tumors progressed during or after chemotherapy. Out of eight evaluable patients, four did not develop WT after 19 weeks of EE4A; four patients developed WT (two while on therapy and two off therapy). The 5-year overall survival was 100% and 6/8 patients achieved bilateral renal preservation.[24]

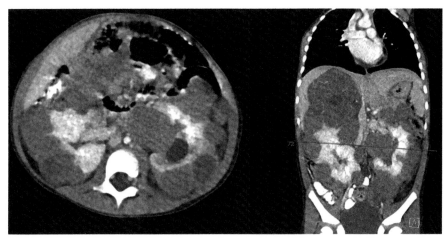

Fig. 4. CT scan demonstrating bilateral, diffuse hyperplastic perilobar nephroblastomatosis.

SUMMARY

Fortunately, the vast majority of children with WT will enjoy good oncologic outcomes. Therefore, future investigation will focus on improving outcomes for patients at increased risk of relapse and decreasing therapy for patients expected to experience excellent results based on risk stratification. From a surgical standpoint, for unilateral WT, a complete upfront resection optimizes disease control and allows for ideal biologic risk stratification. Specifically, surgical education targeting lymph node sampling, both in terms of location and ideal number of nodes to be sampled, will be a major area of study. In addition, surgical intervention can reduce morbidity with the appropriate utilization of post-chemotherapy partial nephrectomy for those children with bilateral WT or unilateral WT with a predisposition syndrome.

CLINICS CARE POINTS

- Wilms tumor is a classic example of a malignancy which requires multimodal therapy and thus multidisciplinary care

DISCLOSURE

No authors have commercial or financial conflicts of interest and no funding sources.

REFERENCES

1. Breslow N, Olshan A, Beckwith JB, et al. Epidemiology of Wilms tumor. Med Pediatr Oncol 1993;21: 172–81.

2. Dome JS, Fernandez CV, Mullen EA, et al. Children's oncology group's 2013 blueprint for research: renal tumors. Pediatr Blood Cancer 2013;60(6):994–1000.

3. Irtan S, Ehrlich PF, Pritchard-Jones K. Wilms tumor: "State-of-the-art" update, 2016. Semin Pediatr Surg 2016;25:250–6.

4. Nakata K, Colombet M, Stiller CA, et al. Incidence of childhood renal tumours: an international population-based study. Int J Cancer 2020;147: 3313–27.

5. Huff V. Wilms' tumours: about tumour suppressor genes, an oncogene and a chameleon gene. Nat Rev Cancer 2011;11:111–21.

6. Saltzman AF. Cost NG: childhood kidney tumors. American Urological Association (AUA) Update Series 2018;37:187–95.

7. Baxter PA, Nuchtern JG, Guillerman RP, et al. Acquired von Willebrand syndrome and Wilms tumor: not always benign. Pediatr Blood Cancer 2009;52: 392–4.

8. Khanna G, Naranjo A, Hoffer F, et al. Detection of preoperative Wilms tumor rupture with CT: a report from the Children's Oncology Group. Radiology 2013;266:610–7.

9. Shamberger RC, Ritchey ML, Haase GM, et al. Intravascular extension of Wilms tumor. Ann Surg 2001; 234:116–21.

10. Ehrlich P, Chi YY, Chintagumpala MM, et al. Results of the first prospective multi-institutional treatment study in children with bilateral Wilms tumor (AREN0534): a report from the children's oncology group. Ann Surg 2017;266:470–8.

11. Qureshi SS, Bhagat M, Kazi M, et al. Standardizing lymph nodal sampling for Wilms tumor: a feasibility study with outcomes. J Pediatr Surg 2020;55: 2668–75.

12. Saltzman AF, Carrasco A Jr, Amini A, et al. Patterns of lymph node sampling and the impact of lymph node density in favorable histology Wilms tumor:

An analysis of the national cancer database. J Pediatr Urol 2018;14:161 e161–161 e168.

13. Saltzman AF, Smith DE, Gao D, et al. How many lymph nodes are enough? Assessing the adequacy of lymph node yield for staging in favorable histology wilms tumor. J Pediatr Surg 2019;54:2331–5.

14. Irtan S, Van Tinteren H, Graf N, et al. Evaluation of needle biopsy as a potential risk factor for local recurrence of Wilms tumour in the SIOP WT 2001 trial. Eur J Cancer 2019;116:13–20.

15. Ritchey M, Daley S, Shamberger RC, et al. Ureteral extension in Wilms' tumor: a report from the National Wilms' Tumor Study Group (NWTSG). J Pediatr Surg 2008;43:1625–9.

16. Fernandez CV, Perlman EJ, Mullen EA, et al. Clinical outcome and biological predictors of relapse after nephrectomy only for very low-risk wilms tumor: a report from children's oncology group AREN0532. Ann Surg 2017;265:835–40.

17. Dix DB, Fernandez CV, Chi YY, et al. Augmentation of therapy for combined loss of heterozygosity 1p and 16q in favorable histology wilms tumor: a children's oncology group AREN0532 and AREN0533 study report. J Clin Oncol 2019;37:2769–77.

18. Fernandez CV, Mullen EA, Chi YY, et al. Outcome and prognostic factors in stage III favorable-histology wilms tumor: a report from the children's oncology group study AREN0532. J Clin Oncol 2018;36:254–61.

19. Dix DB, Seibel NL, Chi YY, et al. Treatment of stage IV favorable histology wilms tumor with lung metastases: a report from the children's oncology group AREN0533 study. J Clin Oncol 2018;36:1564–70.

20. Daw NC, Chi YY, Kim Y, et al. Treatment of stage I anaplastic Wilms' tumour: a report from the Children's Oncology Group AREN0321 study. Eur J Cancer 2019;118:58–66.

21. Daw NC, Chi YY, Kalapurakal JA, et al. Activity of vincristine and irinotecan in diffuse anaplastic wilms tumor and therapy outcomes of stage II to IV disease: results of the children's oncology group AREN0321 study. J Clin Oncol 2020;38:1558–68.

22. Shamberger RC, Haase GM, Argani P, et al. Bilateral Wilms' tumors with progressive or nonresponsive disease. J Pediatr Surg 2006;41:652–7 [discussion: 652-657].

23. Ehrlich PF, Chi YY, Chintagumpala MM, et al. Results of treatment for patients with multicentric or bilaterally predisposed unilateral wilms tumor (AREN0534): a report from the Children's Oncology Group. Cancer 2020;126:3516–25.

24. Ehrlich PF, Tornwall B, Chintagumpala MM, et al. Kidney Preservation and wilms tumor development in children with diffuse hyperplastic perilobar nephroblastomatosis: a report from the children's oncology group study AREN0534. Ann Surg Oncol 2022;29:3252–61.

Pediatric Stone Disease
Current Trends and Future Directions

Ching Man Carmen Tong, DO[a],*, Jonathan S. Ellison, MD[b],
Gregory E. Tasian, MD, MSc, MSCE[c]

KEYWORDS

• Kidney stones • Nephrolithiasis • Children • Calculi • Urolithiasis • Pediatrics

KEY POINTS

- The risk of recurrence for pediatric stone formers is 50% within 3 years of the first symptomatic stone, and those most at risk are adolescents and patients with a prior history of nephrolithiasis.
- Medically complex patients may have several interrelated risk factors for nephrolithiasis, particularly those with alternate routes of nutrition and immobility, warranting a multidisciplinary approach in stone prevention.
- Assessment of a child with suspected kidney stones is similar to that of an adult, although ultrasonography is the preferred initial imaging study, keeping in line with the As Low as Reasonably Achievable principle and the Image Gently Alliance.
- Emerging surgical therapies now focus on minimally invasive approaches for larger stones and reducing radiation exposure with the use of ultrasound-guided endoscopic surgeries instead of fluoroscopy.

BACKGROUND

There has been a rapid increase in the incidence of pediatric nephrolithiasis in the last several decades, with an annual increase of at least 6% to 10%.[1,2] In 2009 alone, an estimated 20 children were hospitalized and more than 90 were treated in the emergency department for urolithiasis daily.[3] A population-based study in South Carolina demonstrated that between 1997 and 2012, the 15- to 19-year-old age group had an observed increased incidence of 26% annually, with a greater increase among females.[4] Although these data reflect a rapid increases in disease incidence from the late 1990s to early 2000s, more contemporary experiences reflect the continued heightened burden of pediatric stone disease.[5] In a nationwide study looking at outpatient management of pediatric upper tract stone disease, the annual expenditure was calculated to be on average $15 million between 2011 and 2018, and this cost increased more over time, reflecting the increase in the prevalence of upper tract stones in children.[6]

The economic burdens and health care costs of pediatric nephrolithiasis are realized partly due to high recurrence rates but also due to complications relating to pain and infections requiring multimodal therapies.[7] The indirect costs and financial impact relating to pediatric urolithiasis may be even greater than what is reported in adult literature, with additional intangible human capital loss such as lost workdays for parents and extra childcare costs if the child misses multiple school days. As the majority of costs were covered by commercial insurance plans as well as government funding, employers and policymakers now have to

[a] Department of Pediatric Urology, University of Alabama at Birmingham, 1600 7th Avenue South, Lowder Suite 318, Birmingham, AL 35233, USA; [b] Department of Urology, Medical College of Wisconsin, Children's Hospital of Wisconsin and Medical College of Wisconsin, 9000 West Wisconsin Avenue, Milwaukee, WI 53226, USA; [c] Division of Urology, Department of Surgery, Children's Hospital of Philadelphia, 3401 Civic Center Boulevard, Philadelphia, PA 19104, USA
* Corresponding author.
E-mail address: carmen.cm.tong@gmail.com

Urol Clin N Am 50 (2023) 465–475
https://doi.org/10.1016/j.ucl.2023.04.009
0094-0143/23/© 2023 Elsevier Inc. All rights reserved.

anticipate increasing health care costs annually with this medical condition.[6]

Because of the overall economic impact, pediatric urologists and nephrologists alike have been working to identify genetic and environmental risk factors pertinent to the pediatric population as well as less invasive techniques to minimize stone burden and recurrence. Herein, the authors review current evidence on risk factors and prevention of stone formation, as well as emerging technologies and surgical interventions on stone treatment pertinent in the pediatric population.

RISK FACTORS
Diet and Fluid Intake

Dietary factors and reduced fluid intake can contribute to metabolic abnormalities and consequently urine supersaturation of calcium, oxalate, and phosphate.[8] There is clear evidence that poor fluid intake and excessive sodium intake, which is prevalent in the Western diet, are two of the most significant risk factors for stone formation.[9] In addition, research has demonstrated that most adolescents and children do not reach adequate fluid intake, and much of the daily intake in their diet is realized from non-water beverages and food moisture.[10] Currently, a randomized controlled trial (PUSH: Prevention of Urinary Stones with Hydration) is being conducted using smart water bottles and smartphone technology to examine the effect of financial incentives and coaching to maintain high fluid intake on the recurrence of symptomatic stones.[11]

Medications

The incidence of drug-induced urolithiasis is about 1% to 2% in the adult population, but there is a paucity of data on the influence of medications in pediatrics.[12] Nonetheless, the mechanisms by which medications can cause pediatric urolithiasis remain the same: either the drug is poorly soluble, leading to filtration of the drug itself into urine and subsequent crystallization, or the drug causes metabolic disturbances that favor urine supersaturation of stone-forming compounds.

One of the most commonly researched classes of medications is antibiotics. Tasian and colleagues performed a large, population-based case-control study from the United Kingdom, using data from more than 600 general practices and more than 13 million children in a span of 10 years.[13] They discovered that cephalosporins, broad-spectrum penicillins, nitrofurantoin, fluoroquinolones, and sulfas were associated with increased chances of nephrolithiasis, even after excluding confounding conditions like urinary tract infections. The odds of nephrolithiasis diminished over time, but were still persistently higher up to 5 years from initial antibiotic administration. The greatest "window of danger" was around 3 to 6 months after exposure to the antibiotic. Children of younger ages were also more susceptible to this association. Typically, these medications precipitate into the urine, crystallize, and obstruct, without causing any metabolic disturbances.[14]

One intriguing theory linking antibiotic usage and nephrolithiasis risk is the impact of these medications on the gut microbiota via a proposed mechanism of changes in macronutrient metabolism from altered composition of the intestinal microbiome.[15] Certainly, gut bacteria is known to be dramatically and persistently reduced even months after the last antibiotic exposure.[16,17] This theory was supported by a case-control study examining the composition of gut microbial communities in patients with known calcium oxalate stone disease.[18] Kidney stone formers were found to have significantly less diverse gut microbiomes, specifically bacteria that produce butyrate and degrade oxalate. Butyrate is responsible for maintaining the gut–mucosal barrier, regulating oxalate transport, and has anti-inflammatory properties; combined with an over-abundance of oxalate from poor degradation, lower production of butyrate may produce the ideal environment for the production of calcium oxalate stones.

Disorders/Anatomic Differences

Patients with malabsorption disorders or a history of urologic reconstructive surgeries with the use of bowel segment, such as augmentation cystoplasty, or urinary stasis due to urologic anomalies or immobility, are at risk for nephrolithiasis. In a study looking at spina bifida individuals after bladder augmentation, approximately 1% of the cohort develop nephrolithiasis annually, with an incidence that is at least 10 times greater than the general population.[19] In particular, those patients were at much greater risk if the augmentation was performed at 10 years of age or older or if they had a prior history of bladder stones. This could be due to the metabolic acidosis that is inherently caused by the use of bowel segment, or mucus generated from the segment itself being refluxed to the kidney and becoming a nidus for stone formation. Other factors that could increase the risks in these patients could include hyperoxaluria due to intestinal malabsorption following bowel resection.

Complex pediatric patients dependent on enteral nutrition are also at higher risk of nephrolithiasis. This may be related to increased sodium and oxalate content and decreased calcium content in tube feeds that predispose the risk of stones.[20] It has also been demonstrated that they have significantly higher levels of urinary oxalate excretion compared to children not on enteral feeds.[21] Further complicating the picture is that many of these patients are also non-ambulatory. Patients who are limited or non-weight bearing may have an increased risk of bone mineral disease and subsequent supersaturation of their urine.[22] In a 10-year study at a tertiary pediatric center, non-ambulatory children were more likely to require surgical interventions for their stones and were more likely to form infection-related stones such as calcium carbonate or struvite stones.[23] Many minimally ambulatory patients also have a component of neurogenic bladder and chronic bacteriuria with urea-splitting organisms, which may explain the propensity for infection-related urolithiasis. The multitude of mechanisms for urinary stone formation in these complex patients highlights the heterogeneity of nephrolithiasis in patients with multiple medical co-morbidities who will often have numerous, interrelated risk factors for stone formation.

EVALUATION

For the most part, evaluation of a symptomatic kidney stone in children is similar to managing a stone episode in an adult. A comprehensive medical history should include information regarding the amount and types of fluid intake, prescription medications, and use of supplements such as vitamins and family history of urolithiasis. Personal history of anatomic disorders of the urinary tract such as ureteropelvic junction obstruction or other disorders that can lead to stone formation such as inflammatory bowel disease should also be ascertained. Older children will have similar presenting symptoms as adults, primarily flank pain, nausea and vomiting, and lower urinary tract symptoms. However, younger or non-communicative patients may not be able to localize pain or articulate their discomfort; in these instances, the medical provider should heavily rely on diagnostic and laboratory testing.

Ultrasonography remains the preferred initial imaging when evaluating children with suspected kidney stones. If a diagnosis cannot be reached from ultrasound alone, then an abdominal plain film or low-dose non-contrast computed tomography (CT) can be performed, particularly in cases with high clinical suspicion. Although critics of ultrasonography will argue that sensitivity of ultrasound is much lower than CT imaging (76% vs near 99%), the lower sensitivity is mostly attributed to missed small non-obstructing stones less than 3 to 4 mm that may otherwise be clinically insignificant and managed conservatively.[24] Sensitivity of ultrasound can further be improved by using adjunctive findings such as presence of ureteral jets and twinkling artifacts under Doppler settings.[25] Given that children are more vulnerable to radiation effects due to increased cell turnover, have a longer life span with greater potential for dose cumulation, and have a higher rate of recurrence than adults, every effort should be made to limit radiation exposure in this population and to follow the principles of ALARA ("As Low as Reasonably Achievable").[26] Therefore, the Image Gently Alliance was launched in 2007 by pediatric radiologists to inform and educate on the use of ionizing radiation when imaging children.[27] Since then, the use of CT imaging in children for evaluation of kidney stones has decreased significantly, such that by 2012, renal ultrasounds became more frequently used than CT.[28,29] Implementation of a clinical care pathway for kidney stones in pediatric emergency departments can also help with decreasing use of CTs, as demonstrated by a study from the Children's Hospital of Philadelphia.[30] This said, CT likely still has a role in situations of a non-diagnostic ultrasound (US) and high clinical suspicion for nephrolithiasis, and in these situations, CT dose modulation efforts should be undertaken.

MEDICAL EXPULSIVE THERAPY

Ureteral stones in children can spontaneously pass about 32% to 63% of the time, so a trial of passage is worth pursuing in the majority of cases, particularly in older children with stones <5 mm in size located in the distal ureter.[31–33] The adjunctive use of medical expulsive therapy with alpha-blockers and calcium-channel blockers has been well-documented for uncomplicated ureteral calculi in adults, and similarly, in children, tamsulosin has now been shown to increase expulsion rate in stones less than 10 mm, regardless of stone size or location.[34,35] To date, there have been six randomized controlled trials examining the role of these medications in children with distal ureteral calculi (**Table 1**).[36–41] A 2022 systematic review and meta-analysis of these six studies demonstrated that the benefits of medical expulsive therapy in children are statistically significant, although only two of these studies were placebo-controlled and none were double-blinded.[42] As well, none of these randomized controlled trials (RCTs) examined the use of calcium-channel blockers.

Table 1
Randomized controlled trials on the role of alpha-blockers in stone passage

Study	Design	Number of Patients	Primary Endpoint	Stone Characteristics	Length of Treatment, Days	Result
Aydogdu et al,[36] 2009 (Turkey, 2009)	Doxazosin (0.03 mg/kg) + ibuprofen vs ibuprofen alone	n = 19 Control = 20	Stone passage confirmed by patient	Distal ureter, <10 mm	21	No difference
Mokhless et al,[37] 2012 (Egypt, 2012)	Tamsulosin (0.2 mg for <5 yo, 0.4 mg for >5 yo) vs ibuprofen	n = 23 Control = 28	Stone passage confirmed by plain film or CT	Distal ureter, <12 mm	28	Improved passage rate with MET, improved time to passage (8.2 vs 14.5 d)
Erturhan et al,[38] 2013 (Turkey, 2013)	Doxazosin (0.03 mg/kg) + ibuprofen vs ibuprofen alone	n = 24 Control = 21	Stone passage confirmed by plain film, ultrasound, or CT	Distal ureter, any size	21	Improved passage rate with MET
Aldaqadossi et al,[39] 2015 (Egypt, 2015)	Tamsulosin (0.2 mg for <5 yo, 0.4 mg for >5 yo) + ibuprofen vs ibuprofen alone	n = 31 Control = 32	Stone passage confirmed by plain film or ultrasound	Distal ureter, <9 mm	28	Improved passage rate with MET
Elgalaly et al,[40] 2017 (Egypt, 2017)	Silodosin (4 mg) vs ibuprofen	n = 20 Control = 19	Stone passage confirmed by plain film or ultrasound	Distal ureter, <10 mm	28	Improved time to passage with MET (7 vs 10 d)
Soliman et al,[41] 2021 (Egypt, 2021)	Silodosin (4 mg) or Tamsulosin 0.4 mg vs placebo	Silodosin, n = 56 Tamsulosin, n = 55 Control = 56	Stone passage by plain film or CT	Distal ureter, <10 mm	28	Silodosin better in passage rate than tamsulosin (89% vs 75%) Tamsulosin better in passage rate than placebo (75% vs 52%)

Abbreviations: CT, computed tomography; MET, medical expulsive therapy.

Nonetheless, current evidence has thus far proved that medical expulsive therapy is safe and effective in children and may help decrease the risk of additional surgery in young children who may have smaller anatomy and increased difficulty navigating the ureter with ureteroscopy. Of note, the use of tamsulosin or alternative alpha-adrenergic antagonists or calcium-channel blockers would be considered 'off-label' use, which should be addressed with the patient and family during counseling. One additional proposed benefit of alpha-blockade is the relaxation of ureteral smooth muscle to facilitate future ureteral access during endoscopy. Preliminary results from McGee and colleagues utilizing preoperative tamsulosin 1 week before surgery suggested that patients who were given preoperative tamsulosin 1 week before surgery had lower rates of failed ureteroscopy.[43] This complementary role of alpha-blockers can potentially decrease the number of trips to the operating room, and in the future, should be an area of focus in clinical and patient outcomes research for pediatric stones.

EMERGING SURGICAL TECHNOLOGIES

There are several anatomic differences unique to children that should be taken into consideration when evaluating for surgery. First, the smaller body habitus and ureteral diameter may make ureteroscopy and use of adult-sized ureteroscopic instruments challenging, especially with primary ureteral access (ie, before ureteral stenting). For these reasons, Ellison and Yonekawa proposed six characteristics of an ideal surgical modality to guide treatment selection: (1) high rate of monotherapeutic success; (2) low risk for complications; (3) ability to return the child to baseline activity; (4) minimized radiation exposure; (5) minimized anesthesia exposure; (6) no need for ancillary procedures.[44]

Patient-centered selection for the ideal surgical modality should include consideration of the patient and stone factors, surgeon experience and resource availability, and perhaps most importantly, patient-driven goals of care. Given the lack of comparative effectiveness data that currently exist within the surgical space of nephrolithiasis, a current patient-centered and expansive observational clinical trial comparing success and patient-reported outcomes across ureteroscopy (URS), shock wave lithotripsy (SWL), and PCNL (the Pediatric KIDnet Stone Care Improvement Network trial— NCT04285658) will complete accrual in May 2023.[45]

A small number of endourology nomograms and scoring systems has recently been developed to predict success rate and surgical outcomes for pediatric patients. There are currently two pediatric nomograms predicting successful treatment with SWL.[46,47] Several studies comparing these two tools have demonstrated that both had good accuracy in their predictions, although the Dogan nomogram had a higher specificity and therefore is considered slightly superior to the Onal nomogram.[48,49] Both scoring systems utilize a combination of gender, age, stone size, and location to predict success, but neither system investigated any correlation with postoperative complications. There are two nomograms for percutaneous nephrolithotomy (PCNL): the stone-kidney size score (SKS) and the Capital Medical University Nomogram (CMUN).[50,51] The SKS only relies on stone-to-kidney size ratio and number of stones and does not factor in staghorn anatomy or location of stones. When comparing it to adult PCNL nomograms, SKS is able to somewhat accurately predict stone-free rate and complications. The CMUN, on the other hand, used data collected from micro and mini PCNL as well as ureteroscopy, and used CT to measure stone burden as opposed to ultrasonography. It has not been externally validated or compared to other nomograms, including the SKS. Because of the heterogeneous data, the CMUN scoring system is more biased and therefore more difficult to generalize and less predictive.

Ureteroscopy is a mainstay for surgical stone treatment, and recent modifications and improved laser technology have made this surgical option even more favored among surgeons. Thulium laser technology was recently introduced in adult endourology and has since been widely adopted after validation of its safety and ease of use.[52] A study from Boston Children's demonstrated improved stone clearance in 109 children with no differences in postoperative complications over 5 years.[53] Although there was no difference in the total operative time in this study, there was a significant difference in laser time, with the longer laser time in the thulium group likely related to low ablation efficiency. Another territory recently explored is ultrasound-guided ureteroscopy, in an effort to decrease radiation exposure during endoscopic surgery. A feasibility study from Morrison and colleagues demonstrated for the first time that laser lithotripsy can be safely performed using ultrasound on patients with lower average BMI.[54] The authors were able to position the ultrasound probe to visualize guidewires, dual-lumen catheters, and ureteroscope throughout the upper urinary tract. Although there would be an expected learning curve to reading real-time ultrasounds intraoperatively, the study offers hope in lowering radiation exposure in these children without compromising stone-free rates or increasing the risk of complications.

New techniques and instrumentation for PCNL have allowed for the use of smaller sheaths, with new techniques named based on the size of the tract: mini (14–24 F), ultra-mini (11–13F), super-mini (10–14F) and even micro (<5F) PCNL.[55] Current evidence has shown the safety and efficacy of these techniques in children regardless of age or size of the stone, with a lower risk of complications for bleeding with smaller sizes.[56,57] A systematic review of micro- and ultra-mini PCNL in children noted that reported stone clearance has ranged from 80% to 100%, with complication rates around 11% to 14%, most relating to extravasation and blood loss with larger tract sizes.[52]

For children with complex medical conditions, contracted body habitus, or ectopically positioned kidneys, conventional approaches with URS, SWL, and PCNL may be challenging. In children who cannot tolerate prone positions or for those with issues related to airway access, the supine PCNL has been successfully performed in children.[58,59] Historically, in situations where endoscopic approaches are not feasible to enable reliable stone clearance, open surgery would be considered. With recent advances in laparoscopic and robotic-assisted techniques, these open approaches have fallen out of favor and perhaps opened additional avenues to consider minimally invasive treatments for upper tract stone disease. Those with complicated renal anatomy such as ureteropelvic junction obstruction requiring pyeloplasty should be considered for robotic surgery for simultaneous nephrolithotomy and upper tract reconstruction.[60,61] Stone clearance in these patients has been shown to be at least 96%.[62]

RECURRENCE AND PREVENTION

In adults, the recurrence rate of a symptomatic stone is 50% within 5 to 10 years of the first episode.[63] In children, this recurrence rate is even more dramatic, with the probability of a recurrent symptomatic stone episode within 3 years.[5] Multiple studies have demonstrated that adolescents and those with a prior history of stone formation are at increased risk for subsequent stone events.[64,65] In a cohort of 200 children from a multi-institutional study, Medairos and colleagues discovered that the incidence of a symptomatic stone event was 41% within 1.5 years and that adolescents had a significantly higher chance of stone events than younger children.[64] They emphasized that this at-risk group in particular should have close follow-up for future stone events. Similarly, results from the Registry for Stones of the Kidney and Ureter also demonstrated that those patients who formed a stone before age 20 are more likely to have recurrent stone events compared to those who formed their first stone later in life.[66]

Ultimately, these patients with a complex disease process should be under multidisciplinary care involving a nutritionist, nephrologist, and urologist. Per American Urological Association (AUA) Guidelines, periodic 24-hour urine studies and basic metabolic panels should be obtained during workup and follow-up of recurrent stone formers and interested first-time stone patients.[67] However, the utility of a full metabolic evaluation with a serum chemistry panel and 24-hour urine studies in a first-time pediatric stone former remains controversial. Although completion of 24-hour urine studies has been shown to help with decreased recurrence of future symptomatic stones, it is expensive, difficult to perform correctly in children with adequate volume, and oftentimes does not lead to increased compliance to prescribed treatments.[68] In a study of 800 patients at a high-volume tertiary care center, nearly 50% completed a 24-hour urine study, which admittedly is higher than reported literature.[69] Those who were older in age, who had renal colic with first stone presentation, and who had a family history of stones were more likely to complete the 24-hour urine analyses, but those on government-subsidized insurance were less likely.

Preventive measures should first focus on risk factors that are modifiable. Increasing fluid intake is often the first step in prevention.[70] This is particularly important in patients who live in hot climates or during the summer months when children are more likely to play outdoors in the sun. In a study looking at drinking behaviors in adolescents and response to fluid intake during school, it was noted that this age group is particularly unaware of their daily water intake and is also slow to respond to thirst.[71] Although there is no consensus on how much fluid intake is appropriate for prevention, some base their recommendations on daily urine volumes: infants should maintain a volume greater than 750 mL, children younger than 5 should have greater than 1000 mL, those between 5 and 10 years old should have greater than 1500 mL, and adolescents should aim for greater than 2 L.[72] Researchers have also used 24-h urine collections to develop an equation to help achieve increased urine output goals in adolescents with stones.[73] This equation, known as the fluid prescription, determines the additional fluid intake needed to produce the desired increase in urine output by dividing the desired urine output by

Table 2
Dietary recommendations and weight-based medications for selective metabolic abnormalities

Metabolic Abnormality	Dietary Changes	Pharmaceutical Therapies	Mechanism of Action	Side Effects	FDA-Approved?
Hypocitraturia	Increase potassium- and citrate-rich vegetables and fruits, such as pineapples, tomatoes, bananas	Potassium citrate 2–4 mEq/kg/d	Raises urine pH by providing an alkali load; raises urine citrate excretion	Hyperkalemia, GI discomfort (nausea, diarrhea, vomiting)	Off-label
Hypercalciuria	Low-sodium diet <2 g/d	Hydrochlorothiazide 1–2 mg/kg/d, up to 25–50 mg daily Chlorthalidone initial 0.3 mg/kg/d, up to 2 mg/kg/d or 50 mg/d	Promotes release of sodium into urine and reabsorption of calcium	Hypokalemia, hyponatremia, hypercalcemia	Off-label
Hyperuricosuria	Decrease non-dairy protein and sodium	Allopurinol 4–10 mg/kg/d	Lowers serum and urine uric acid (xanthine oxidase inhibitor)	Hepatotoxicity, delayed hypersensitivity reactions (Stevens-Johnson syndrome)	Off-label
Cystinuria	Decrease sodium intake Higher fluid intake	Alpha-mercaptopropionyl glycine (tiopronin)	Increases solubility of cystine	Fatigue, rash, oral mucosal ulcers, GI discomfort (nausea, diarrhea)	Yes
Hyperoxaluria	Limit daily oxalate Maintain high calcium intake	Lumasiran (for primary hyperoxaluria type 1) Calcium supplementation for enteric hyperoxaluria	Reduces levels of glycolate oxidase enzyme, which reduces the amount of glyoxylate (substrate for oxalate production)	Injection site reaction, abdominal pain	Yes

0.71. For instance, if a child, based on their urine collection results, needs to increase their 24-hour urine output by 500 cc to reach a goal of 2 L, then the recommended increase in the daily fluid intake is 704 mL. Children should also aim for a low-sodium diet and a healthy daily number of citrate-heavy fruits and vegetables. Restriction on animal protein intake is usually not indicated and may adversely affect the linear growth and development of young children. Additionally, as calcium reduction paradoxically increases stone risk and may negatively impact bone health and development, moderate calcium intake is recommended. If dietary changes are not sufficient, pharmacologic therapies may be necessary to decrease recurrence (**Table 2**).

SUMMARY

Pediatric nephrolithiasis is now a public health burden and a looming crisis due to the meteoric increase in incidence within the last several decades. A significant effort in the research community has thus focused on identifying modifiable risk factors, such as environmental exposures, dietary contributors, and effects of medications on gut microbiome, to help educate the medical community and the public on the prevention of stones. We now know that children have a 50% chance of a recurrent stone episode within 3 years. We also know that adolescents and those with complex chronic medical conditions are particularly vulnerable to kidney stone formation. Careful selection of management therapies with a strong emphasis on preventive measures is essential in curbing recurrent stone episodes in pediatric patients, and future research should focus on minimally invasive surgical techniques that minimize ionizing radiation and repeated exposure to general anesthesia.

CLINICS CARE POINTS

- The risk of recurrence for pediatric stone formers is 50% within 3 years of first symptomatic stone, and those most at risk are adolescents and patients with prior history of nephrolithiasis.
- Medically complex patients may have several interrelated risk factors for nephrolithiasis, particularly those with alternate routes of nutrition and immobility, warranting a multidisciplinary approach in stone prevention.
- Assessment of a child with suspected kidney stones is similar to that of an adult, although ultrasonography is the preferred initial imaging study, keeping in line with the ALARA principle and the Image Gently Alliance.
- Emerging surgical therapies now focus on minimally invasive approaches for larger stones and reducing radiation exposure with use of ultrasound-guided endoscopic surgeries instead of fluoroscopy.

FINANCIAL DISCLOSURES

C.M. Carmen Tong has no conflicts of interest or financial disclosures. J.S. Ellison is a consultant to Alnylam Pharmaceuticals and a contributor to UpToDate. G.E. Tasian is on the scientific advisory board for Alnylam and NovoNordisk.

REFERENCES

1. Sas DJ, Hulsey TC, Shatat IF, et al. Increasing Incidence of Kidney Stones in Children Evaluated in the Emergency Department. J Pediatr 2010;157. https://doi.org/10.1016/j.jpeds.2010.02.004. Epub ahead of print.
2. Routh JC, Graham DA, Nelson CP. Epidemiological trends in pediatric urolithiasis at United States freestanding pediatric hospitals. J Urol 2010;184. https://doi.org/10.1016/j.juro.2010.05.018. Epub ahead of print.
3. Wang HHS, Wiener JS, Lipkin ME, et al. Estimating the nationwide, hospital based economic impact of pediatric urolithiasis. J Urol 2015;193. https://doi.org/10.1016/j.juro.2014.09.116. Epub ahead of print.
4. Tasian GE, Ross ME, Song L, et al. Annual incidence of nephrolithiasis among children and adults in South Carolina from 1997 to 2012. Clin J Am Soc Nephrol 2016;11. https://doi.org/10.2215/CJN.07610715. Epub ahead of print.
5. Tasian GE, Kabarriti AE, Kalmus A, et al. Kidney Stone Recurrence among Children and Adolescents. J Urol 2017;197. https://doi.org/10.1016/j.juro.2016.07.090. Epub ahead of print.
6. Sturgis MR, Becerra AZ, Khusid JA, et al. The monetary costs of pediatric upper urinary tract stone disease: Analysis in a contemporary United States cohort. J Pediatr Urol 2022;18. https://doi.org/10.1016/j.jpurol.2022.02.019. Epub ahead of print.
7. Roberson D, Sperling C, Shah A, et al. Economic Considerations in the Management of Nephrolithiasis. Curr Urol Rep 2020;21. https://doi.org/10.1007/s11934-020-00971-6. Epub ahead of print.
8. Bowen DK, Tasian GE. Pediatric Stone Disease Pediatrics Urology Nephrolithiasis Diagnostic imaging Medical management. Urologic Clinics of NA 2022;45:539–50.

9. Ciongradi CI, Filip F, Sârbu I, et al. The Impact of Water and Other Fluids on Pediatric Nephrolithiasis. Nutrients 2022;14:1–10.

10. Kant AK, Graubard BI. Contributors of water intake in US children and adolescents: associations with dietary and meal characteristics - National Health and Nutrition Examination Survey 2005-2006. Am J Clin Nutr 2010;92. https://doi.org/10.3945/ajcn.2010.29708. Epub ahead of print.

11. Scales CD, Desai AC, Harper JD, et al. Prevention of Urinary Stones With Hydration (PUSH): Design and Rationale of a Clinical Trial. Am J Kidney Dis 2021; 77. https://doi.org/10.1053/j.ajkd.2020.09.016. Epub ahead of print.

12. Daudon M, Frochot V, Bazin D, et al. Drug-induced kidney stones and crystalline nephropathy: Pathophysiology, prevention and treatment. Drugs 2018;78. https://doi.org/10.1007/s40265-017-0853-7. Epub ahead of print.

13. Tasian GE, Jemielita T, Goldfarb DS, et al. Oral antibiotic exposure and kidney stone disease. J Am Soc Nephrol 2018;29. https://doi.org/10.1681/ASN.2017111213. Epub ahead of print.

14. Sighinolfi MC, Eissa A, Bevilacqua L, et al. Drug-Induced Urolithiasis in Pediatric Patients. Pediatr Drugs 2019;21. https://doi.org/10.1007/s40272-019-00355-5. Epub ahead of print.

15. Cox LM, Yamanishi S, Sohn J, et al. Altering the intestinal microbiota during a critical developmental window has lasting metabolic consequences. Cell 2014;158. https://doi.org/10.1016/j.cell.2014.05.052. Epub ahead of print.

16. Kelly JP, Curhan GC, Cave DR, et al. Factors related to colonization with oxalobacter formigenes in U.S. Adults. J Endourol 2011;25. https://doi.org/10.1089/end.2010.0462. Epub ahead of print.

17. Dethlefsen L, Huse S, Sogin ML, et al. The pervasive effects of an antibiotic on the human gut microbiota, as revealed by deep 16s rRNA sequencing. PLoS Biol 2008;6. https://doi.org/10.1371/journal.pbio.0060280. Epub ahead of print.

18. Denburg MR, Koepsell K, Lee JJ, et al. Perturbations of the gut microbiome and metabolome in children with calcium oxalate kidney stone disease. J Am Soc Nephrol 2020;31. https://doi.org/10.1681/ASN.2019101131. Epub ahead of print.

19. Salama AK, Misseri R, Hollowell N, et al. Incidence of nephrolithiasis after bladder augmentation in people with spina bifida. J Pediatr Urol 2021;17. https://doi.org/10.1016/j.jpurol.2021.03.012. Epub ahead of print.

20. Pozzi M, Locatelli F, Galbiati S, et al. Relationships between enteral nutrition facts and urinary stones in a cohort of pediatric patients in rehabilitation from severe acquired brain injury. Clin Nutr 2019;38. https://doi.org/10.1016/j.clnu.2018.05.005. Epub ahead of print.

21. DeFoor W, Nehus E, Schulte M, et al. Enteral nutrition and the risk of nephrolithiasis in complex pediatric patients. J Pediatr Urol 2022;18:743.e1–6.

22. Schwaderer AL, Oduguwa A, Kusumi K. Urinary stone disease in pediatric and adult metabolic bone clinic patients. Urolithiasis 2018;46. https://doi.org/10.1007/s00240-017-0968-z. Epub ahead of print.

23. Hannallah A, Baker ZG, Bajakian T, et al. Nephrolithiasis management and outcomes in pediatric patients with limited mobility. J Pediatr Urol 2022;18:585.e1–7.

24. Passerotti C, Chow JS, Silva A, et al. Ultrasound versus computerized tomography for evaluating urolithiasis. J Urol 2009. https://doi.org/10.1016/j.juro.2009.03.072. Epub ahead of print.

25. Sahadev R, Maxon V, Srinivasan A. Approaches to Eliminate Radiation Exposure in the Management of Pediatric Urolithiasis. Curr Urol Rep 2018;19. https://doi.org/10.1007/s11934-018-0832-x. Epub ahead of print.

26. Kaste S. TH-D-BRA-04: Late Effects from Diagnostic Imaging. Med Phys 2010. https://doi.org/10.1118/1.3469537. Epub ahead of print 2010.

27. Frush DP, Strauss KJ. Image Gently: Getting It Right. J Am Coll Radiol 2017;14. https://doi.org/10.1016/j.jacr.2017.02.052. Epub ahead of print.

28. Streur CS, Lin PJ, Hollingsworth JM, et al. Pediatric Urology Impact of the Image Gently Ò Campaign on Computerized Tomography Use for Evaluation of Pediatric Nephrolithiasis. J Urol 2019;201:996–1004.

29. Menoch MJA, Hirsh DA, Khan NS, et al. Trends in computed tomography utilization in the pediatric emergency department. Pediatrics 2012;129. https://doi.org/10.1542/peds.2011-2548. Epub ahead of print.

30. Ziemba JB, Canning DA, Lavelle J, et al. Patient and institutional characteristics associated with initial computerized tomography in children presenting to the emergency department with kidney stones. J Urol 2015;193. https://doi.org/10.1016/j.juro.2014.09.115. Epub ahead of print.

31. Pietrow PK, Pope IVJC, Adams MC, et al. Clinical outcome of pediatric stone disease. J Urol 2002; 167. https://doi.org/10.1097/00005392-200202000-00060. Epub ahead of print.

32. Kalorin CM, Zabinski A, Okpareke I, et al. Pediatric Urinary Stone Disease-Does Age Matter? J Urol 2009;181. https://doi.org/10.1016/j.juro.2009.01.050. Epub ahead of print.

33. Dangle P, Ayyash O, Shaikh H, et al. Predicting spontaneous stone passage in prepubertal children: A single institution cohort. J Endourol 2016;30. https://doi.org/10.1089/end.2015.0565. Epub ahead of print.

34. Assimos D, Krambeck A, Miller NL, et al. Surgical Management of Stones: American Urological

Association/Endourological Society Guideline, PART I. J Urol 2016;196. https://doi.org/10.1016/j.juro.2016.05.090. Epub ahead of print.

35. Tasian GE, Cost NG, Granberg CF, et al. Tamsulosin and spontaneous passage of ureteral stones in children: A multi-institutional cohort study. J Urol 2014;192. https://doi.org/10.1016/j.juro.2014.01.091. Epub ahead of print.

36. Aydogdu O, Burgu B, Gucuk A, et al. Effectiveness of Doxazosin in Treatment of Distal Ureteral Stones in Children. J Urol 2009;182. https://doi.org/10.1016/j.juro.2009.08.061. Epub ahead of print.

37. Mokhless I, Zahran AR, Youssif M, et al. Tamsulosin for the management of distal ureteral stones in children: A prospective randomized study. J Pediatr Urol 2012;8. https://doi.org/10.1016/j.jpurol.2011.09.008. Epub ahead of print.

38. Erturhan S, Bayrak O, Sarica K, et al. Efficacy of medical expulsive treatment with doxazosin in pediatric patients. Urology 2013;81. https://doi.org/10.1016/j.urology.2012.11.031. Epub ahead of print.

39. Aldaqadossi HA, Shaker H, Saifelnasr M, et al. Efficacy and safety of tamsulosin as a medical expulsive therapy for stones in children. Arab J Urol 2015;13. https://doi.org/10.1016/j.aju.2015.02.007. Epub ahead of print.

40. Elgalaly H, Eliwa A, Seleem M, et al. Silodosin in the treatment of distal ureteric stones in children: A prospective, randomised, placebo-controlled study. Arab J Urol 2017;15. https://doi.org/10.1016/j.aju.2017.05.005. Epub ahead of print.

41. Soliman MG, El-Gamal O, El-Gamal S, et al. Silodosin versus Tamsulosin as Medical Expulsive Therapy for Children with Lower-Third Ureteral Stones: Prospective Randomized Placebo-Controlled Study. Urol Int 2021;105. https://doi.org/10.1159/000513074. Epub ahead of print.

42. Bacchus MW, Locke RA, Kwenda EP, et al. Medical Expulsive Therapy (MET) for Ureteral Calculi in Children: Systematic Review and Meta-Analysis. Frontiers in Urology 2022;2:1–8.

43. McGee LM, Sack BS, Wan J, et al. The effect of preoperative tamsulosin on ureteroscopic access in school-aged children. J Pediatr Urol 2021;17. https://doi.org/10.1016/j.jpurol.2021.08.021. Epub ahead of print.

44. Ellison JS, Yonekawa K. Recent Advances in the Evaluation, Medical, and Surgical Management of Pediatric Nephrolithiasis. Current Pediatrics Reports 2018;6. https://doi.org/10.1007/s40124-018-0176-5. Epub ahead of print.

45. Ellison JS, Lorenzo M, Beck H, et al. Comparative effectiveness of paediatric kidney stone surgery (the PKIDS trial): Study protocol for a patient-centred pragmatic clinical trial. BMJ Open 2022;12. https://doi.org/10.1136/bmjopen-2021-056789. Epub ahead of print.

46. Dogan HS, Altan M, Citamak B, et al. A new nomogram for prediction of outcome of pediatric shock-wave lithotripsy. J Pediatr Urol 2015;11. https://doi.org/10.1016/j.jpurol.2015.01.004. Epub ahead of print.

47. Onal B, Tansu N, Demirkesen O, et al. Nomogram and scoring system for predicting stone-free status after extracorporeal shock wave lithotripsy in children with urolithiasis. BJU Int 2013;111. https://doi.org/10.1111/j.1464-410X.2012.11281.x. Epub ahead of print.

48. Brown G, Juliebø-Jones P, Keller EX, et al. Current status of nomograms and scoring systems in paediatric endourology: A systematic review of literature. J Pediatr Urol 2022;18:572–84.

49. Ceyhan E, Ozer C, Ozturk B, et al. Ability of ESWL nomograms to predict stone-free rate in children. J Pediatr Urol 2021;17. https://doi.org/10.1016/j.jpurol.2021.03.025. Epub ahead of print.

50. Çitamak B, Dogan HS, Ceylan T, et al. A new simple scoring system for prediction of success and complication rates in pediatric percutaneous nephrolithotomy: stone-kidney size score. J Pediatr Urol 2019;15. https://doi.org/10.1016/j.jpurol.2018.09.019. Epub ahead of print.

51. Zhang Y, Li J, Zhang D, et al. Nomograms predicting the outcomes of endoscopic treatments for pediatric upper urinary tract calculi. Int J Urol 2021;28. https://doi.org/10.1111/iju.14451. Epub ahead of print.

52. Jones P, Bennett G, Aboumarzouk OM, et al. Role of Minimally Invasive Percutaneous Nephrolithotomy Techniques - Micro and Ultra-Mini PCNL (<15F) in the Pediatric Population: A Systematic Review. J Endourol 2017;31. https://doi.org/10.1089/end.2017.0136. Epub ahead of print.

53. Jaeger CD, Nelson CP, Cilento BG, et al. Comparing Pediatric Ureteroscopy Outcomes with SuperPulsed Thulium Fiber Laser and Low-Power Holmium:YAG Laser. J Urol 2022;208:426–33.

54. Morrison JC, van Batavia JP, Darge K, et al. Ultrasound guided ureteroscopy in children: Safety and success. J Pediatr Urol 2018;14. https://doi.org/10.1016/j.jpurol.2017.08.019. Epub ahead of print.

55. Proietti S, Giusti G, Desai M, et al. A Critical Review of Miniaturised Percutaneous Nephrolithotomy: Is Smaller Better? Eur Urol Foc 2017;3. https://doi.org/10.1016/j.euf.2017.05.001. Epub ahead of print.

56. Mahmood SN, Falah B, Ahmed C, et al. Is Mini Percutaneous Nephrolithotomy a Game Changer for the Treatment of Renal Stones in Children? Eur Urol Open Sci 2022;37. https://doi.org/10.1016/j.euros.2021.12.014. Epub ahead of print.

57. Celik H, Camtosun A, Altintas R, et al. Percutaneous nephrolithotomy in children with pediatric and adult-sized instruments. J Pediatr Urol 2016;12. https://doi.org/10.1016/j.jpurol.2016.04.053. Epub ahead of print.

58. Desoky EAE, Sakr AM, Elsayed ER, et al. Ultra-Mini-Percutaneous Nephrolithotomy in Flank-Free

Modified Supine Position vs Prone Position in Treatment of Pediatric Renal Pelvic and Lower Caliceal Stones. J Endourol 2022;36. https://doi.org/10.1089/end.2021.0557. Epub ahead of print.

59. Softness KA, Kurtz MP. Pediatric Stone Surgery: What Is Hot and What Is Not. Curr Urol Rep 2022; 23. https://doi.org/10.1007/s11934-022-01089-7. Epub ahead of print.

60. Borofsky MS, Lingeman JE. The role of open and laparoscopic stone surgery in the modern era of endourology. Nat Rev Urol 2015;12. https://doi.org/10.1038/nrurol.2015.141. Epub ahead of print.

61. Peng T, Zhong H, Hu B, et al. Minimally invasive surgery for pediatric renal and ureteric stones: A therapeutic update. Front Pediatr 2022;10. https://doi.org/10.3389/fped.2022.902573. Epub ahead of print.

62. Swearingen R, Sood A, Madi R, et al. Zero-fragment Nephrolithotomy: A Multi-center Evaluation of Robotic Pyelolithotomy and Nephrolithotomy for Treating Renal Stones. Eur Urol 2017;72. https://doi.org/10.1016/j.eururo.2016.10.021. Epub ahead of print.

63. Ljunghall S, Danielson BG. A Prospective Study of Renal Stone Recurrences. Br J Urol 1984;56. https://doi.org/10.1111/j.1464-410X.1984.tb05346.x. Epub ahead of print.

64. Medairos R, Paloian NJ, Pan A, et al. Risk factors for subsequent stone events in pediatric nephrolithiasis: A multi-institutional analysis. J Pediatr Urol 2022;18. https://doi.org/10.1016/j.jpurol.2021.11.012. Epub ahead of print.

65. Ferraro PM, Curhan GC, D'Addessi A, et al. Risk of recurrence of idiopathic calcium kidney stones: analysis of data from the literature. J Nephrol 2017; 30. https://doi.org/10.1007/s40620-016-0283-8. Epub ahead of print.

66. Li Y, Bayne D, Wiener S, et al. Stone formation in patients less than 20 years of age is associated with higher rates of stone recurrence: Results from the Registry for Stones of the Kidney and Ureter (ReSKU). J Pediatr Urol 2020;16. https://doi.org/10.1016/j.jpurol.2020.03.014. Epub ahead of print.

67. Pearle MS, Goldfarb DS, Assimos DG, et al. Medical management of kidney stones: AUA guideline. J Urol 2014;192. https://doi.org/10.1016/j.juro.2014.05.006. Epub ahead of print.

68. Carnes K, Howe A, Feustel PJ, et al. 24-Hour urine collection for first time pediatric stone formers: Is it worth it? J Pediatr Urol 2021;17. https://doi.org/10.1016/j.jpurol.2020.12.001. Epub ahead of print.

69. Lee AS, McGarry L, Bowen DK, et al. Patient Characteristics Associated With Completion of 24-hour Urine Analyses Among Children and Adolescents With Nephrolithiasis. Urology 2019;127. https://doi.org/10.1016/j.urology.2019.02.008. Epub ahead of print.

70. Hernandez JD, Ellison JS, Lendvay TS. Current trends, evaluation, and management of pediatric nephrolithiasis. JAMA Pediatr 2015;169. https://doi.org/10.1001/jamapediatrics.2015.1419. Epub ahead of print.

71. Tasian GE, Ross M, Song L, et al. Ecological momentary assessment of factors associated with water intake among adolescents with kidney stone disease. J Urol 2019;201. https://doi.org/10.1016/j.juro.2018.07.064. Epub ahead of print.

72. Edvardsson VO, Goldfarb DS, Lieske JC, et al. Hereditary causes of kidney stones and chronic kidney disease. Pediatr Nephrol 2013;28. https://doi.org/10.1007/s00467-012-2329-z. Epub ahead of print.

73. Bernard J, Song L, Henderson B, et al. Association Between Daily Water Intake and 24-hour Urine Volume Among Adolescents With Kidney Stones. Urology 2020;140. https://doi.org/10.1016/j.urology.2020.01.024. Epub ahead of print.

Diagnosis, Classification, and Contemporary Management of Undescended Testicles

Emily R. Chedrawe, MD[a,b], Daniel T. Keefe, MD, MSc[a,b],
Rodrigo L.P. Romao, MD MSc[a,b,c],*

KEYWORDS

- Cryptorchidism • Undescended testicle • Orchidopexy • Fowler-Stephens • Fertility
- Testis cancer

KEY POINTS

- Undescended testicles are a common congenital anomaly in male patients with a prevalence of 1% to 2%, which has remained stable over time.
- This condition is a risk factor for infertility and testicular cancer.
- Diagnosis is based on physical examination findings and imaging is unnecessary in routine cases of undescended testicles.
- Surgical fixation is the mainstay of treatment and may include different approaches (inguinal, pre-scrotal, or laparoscopic) depending on physical examination findings.

INTRODUCTION

Undescended testis (UDT), or cryptorchidism, is the absence of the testis in the normal scrotal position, defined as a testicle at or below the mid-scrotum.[1] UDT is a common condition in male patients often noted at birth but can be identified in older patients. The etiology of UDT is complex with multifactorial causes related to the interplay of the environment, genetics, and hormones. Physical examination is the mainstay of diagnosis and, in routine cases, imaging modalities are not required before proceeding with treatment. In complex cases where there are bilateral unde-scended testicles, especially nonpalpable testes (NPT), or there is an association with hypospadias, consideration of a difference of sexual differentia-tion (DSD) is important and urgent consultation with specialists is warranted.

UDT represents a risk factor for future infertility and testicular malignancy, which are the main rea-sons for concern for families of patients with this condition. This article highlights the clinician's role in providing evidence-based counseling regarding both the short-term and long-term out-comes of UDT. Herein, we provide a summary of the epidemiology, classification, long-term risks, clinical presentation, and surgical treatment of UDT.

ETIOLOGY

The etiology of UDT requires an understanding of testicular embryologic development. The testes develop within the abdomen and descend through the inguinal canal to the scrotum in a trajectory determined by the gubernaculum.[2] Testicular descent occurs in 2 stages. After sexual

[a] Division of Pediatric Urology, IWK Health Centre, 5850 University Avenue, P.O. Box 9700, Halifax, NS, B3K 6R8 Canada; [b] Department of Urology, Dalhousie University, 1276 South Park Street. Room 293, 5 Victoria, Halifax, NS, B3H 2Y9, Canada; [c] Division of Pediatric Surgery and Department of Surgery, IWK Health Centre, Dalhousie University, 5850 University Avenue, P.O. Box 9700, Halifax, NS, B3K 6R8
* Corresponding author. Division of Pediatric Urology, IWK Health Centre, 5850 University Avenue, P.O. Box 9700, Halifax, NS, B3K 6R8.
E-mail address: rodrigo.lp.romao@gmail.com

Urol Clin N Am 50 (2023) 477–490
https://doi.org/10.1016/j.ucl.2023.04.011

differentiation the testes remain in an intra-abdominal location until 25 to 28 weeks gestation, when descent into the inguinal canal begins. The final scrotal position is not met until the third trimester of gestation or soon after birth.[2,3] The cause of cryptorchidism is not completely understood but thought to be a combination of genetic and environmental factors.[4]

CLASSIFICATION

The classification of UDT is based on the clinical examination findings, age of presentation, and intraoperative findings. It is important to distinguish whether the condition is unilateral or bilateral. The most commonly recognized diagnostic entities are summarized in **Table 1** and include the following:

Congenital versus Acquired

Congenital UDT refers to a testis that is not identified in the scrotum at birth, whereas acquired UDT refers to a testis palpated in the normal scrotal position at birth but later found to be extra-scrotal. Ascending testes were reliably documented to be in the scrotum early in life but currently do not reach a scrotal position comfortably on physical examination.[5] Ascending testis is often considered acquired cryptorchidism because the testis is present in the normal scrotal position at birth and then migrates. A small proportion of retractile testes can become ascending testes over time.

Retractile testis represents a testicle that can intermittently ascend out of the normal scrotal position related to a brisk cremasteric reflex but can be manipulated back and remains in a scrotal position for at least a few seconds, until stimulation causes them to retract again. Retractile testes are not considered UDT although they should be monitored due to the risk of becoming an ascending testicle over time, which happens in approximately 10% to 30% of cases.[6]

Palpable versus Nonpalpable

Palpable testicles are those that are identified on clinical examination but are not located in the dependent portion of the scrotum. An UDT is usually found anywhere along the normal path of descent, such as abdominal (proximal to internal inguinal ring, near the iliac vessels, or kidney), or canalicular (within the inguinal canal). A testis outside this expected trajectory of descent through the ipsilateral inguinal canal is considered an ectopic testis. The most common location for an ectopic testicle is the superficial inguinal pouch (anterior to the external oblique fascia). Other ectopic locations include the following: perirenal, prepubic (medial to the external ring), femoral, peripenile, perineal, or contralateral scrotal (**Fig. 1**).[7]

NPT are defined as the inability to palpate the testicle during examination. In this case, the diagnosis could include an intra-abdominal testis, ectopic testis, vanishing testis, testicular agenesis, or an inaccurate examination. Vanishing testis is a term used to explain a proposed phenomenon where the testis is present during development but thought to be absent at birth due to a vascular accident or torsion.[8] When this occurs, the surgeon may identify a small residual amount of tissue known as a testicular nubbin. This is most commonly a unilateral event (monorchia) but can rarely be bilateral resulting in anorchia. Agenesis refers to a testis that never developed in the first place.

EPIDEMIOLOGY

The incidence of UDT is variable and associated with gestational age. An epidemiologic systematic review reports a prevalence in full term male neonates of 1.0% to 4.6% compared with 1.1% to 45.3% of preterm/low birth weight male neonates.[9] The incidence of UDT decreases to approximately 1.0% at 1 year of age after allowing time for spontaneous descent, which has been estimated at 35% to 43% in some studies.[10–12] Descent is most likely to occur within 3 months after birth in full-term boys.

A Canadian regional population study observing rates of cryptorchidism more than 26 years showed the prevalence of UDT has remained stable over time. Our group identified clustering of UDT cases in counties associated with intense agricultural activity, a phenomenon that was not observed for other, nonendocrine-mediated congenital malformations.[13] However, a more granular follow-up study at the postal code level did not confirm that pattern.[14]

Most cases of UDT are sporadic with up to 85% of cases considered nonsyndromic; however, cryptorchidism has been associated with hundreds of syndromes involving more than 300 genes. Bilateral cryptorchidism is found in about 10% of cases.[15] The prevalence of UDT and the different classifications varies across studies due to diverse definitions. A majority, approximately 62% to 75%, of UDT are congenital, palpable, and unilateral, whereas approximately 20% are NPT.[9] Within the classification of NPT, intra-abdominal testes are found in approximately 10% of boys with UDT, and 4% represent vanishing testis.[16,17]

Table 1
Classification and definition of undescended testis

Classification	Definition	Congenital vs Acquired	Palpable vs Nonpalpable	Frequency of UDT
Suprascrotal	Above the midscrotal position and below the external inguinal ring	Either	Palpable	15% of UDT
Inguinal	Palpated or surgically located within the inguinal canal. Also referred to as canalicular	Either	Palpable	Up to 80% of UDT
Abdominal	Proximal to the internal inguinal ring, near the iliac vessels or kidney	Congenital	Nonpalpable	10% of all UDT
Ectopic	Found outside the expected trajectory of descent	Congenital	Either	About 4% of all UDT
Vanishing testis	Often represents a testicle present during development but absent at birth—from a possible vascular accident or torsion. Usually a nubbin can be identified in the inguinal or scrotal position	Congenital	Nubbin may be palpable	<5% of all UDT
Agenesis	A testis that did not develop	Congenital	Nonpalpable	<5% of all UDT
Ascending testis	Documented in the normal scrotal position but then migrates	Acquired	Usually palpable	1.5% of prepubertal boys
Iatrogenic	Previous inguinal surgery—often infant inguinal hernia repair. Testis gets trapped in scar tissue. Typically found in the inguinal canal	Acquired	Usually palpable	2% after inguinal hernia repair, 10% after primary inguinal orchidopexy

(continued on next page)

Table 1 (continued)				
Classification	Definition	Congenital vs Acquired	Palpable vs Nonpalpable	Frequency of UDT
Retractile testis	Not considered UDT—but can progress to ascending testis Testicle that intermittently ascends from the normal scrotal position related to a brisk cremasteric reflex but can be manipulated back to a normal position and remain for at least a few seconds	-	Palpable	30% of prepubertal boys, decreases to 4% at age 12

Acquired cryptorchidism, or ascending testes related to ascension of previously documented retractile testes, are less common and found in only 1.5% of prepubertal boys. With development, there is a decrease in the reported incidence of retractile testes with an estimated rate of 30% of boys aged 4 years and only 4% of boys aged 12 years.[18] Ascending testes are typically found unilaterally and distal to the inguinal ring either in the prescrotal, superficial inguinal pouch or in the high scrotal position. The detection of acquired cryptorchidism is important because these patients can have similar histologic changes as seen in congenital cases.[19] Another cause of acquired cryptorchidism is previous inguinal surgery, particularly inguinal hernia repair in infants, where the testis was not properly manipulated back to the scrotum at the end of the case. It is usually found "trapped" in scar tissue in the inguinal canal.[20]

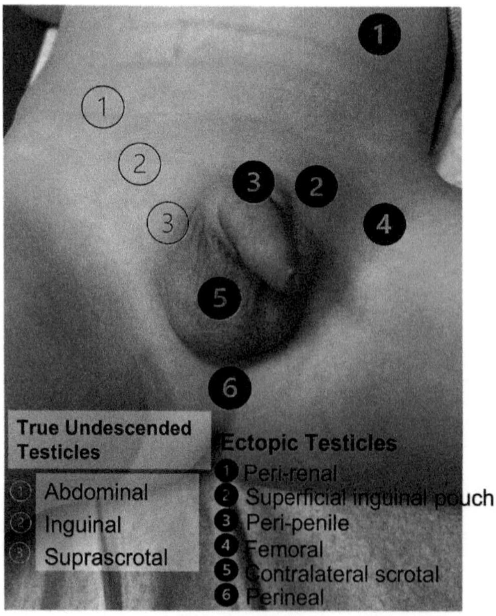

Ectopic testis is a less common form of cryptorchidism and thought to be a failure in the second portion of testicular descent where the testis does not migrate through the external inguinal ring.[21,22] Similar histopathology is noted in ectopic and UDT suggesting ectopic testes are a product of aberrant migration as opposed to endocrinopathy.[22] Although research is limited, a more recent study found the incidence of testicular ectopia was 3.9% out of 1132 patients with UDT.[7] The most common location of a testis outside of the path of normal descent is the superficial inguinal (Dennis-Browne) pouch followed by the perineum (1% of all UDT, 33% of ectopic testis), femoral canal (19%), contralateral scrotum (14%), and peri-penile region (14%).[7,23]

Fig. 1. Potential undescended and ectopic testis locations in cryptorchidism.

True Undescended Testicles
1 Abdominal
2 Inguinal
3 Suprascrotal

Ectopic Testicles
1 Peri-renal
2 Superficial inguinal pouch
3 Peri-penile
4 Femoral
5 Contralateral scrotal
6 Perineal

EVIDENCE-BASED ASSESSMENT OF RISK FOR LONG-TERM MORBIDITY

Our current knowledge about the long-term morbidity of cryptorchidism is limited because studies in this area are challenging due to the need for long-term follow-up, inconsistencies in classification and age of diagnosis, and variability in timing and type of intervention. The morbidity of cryptorchidism is likely associated with the location of the UDT and the age of intervention.

Fertility Issues

Cryptorchidism affects fertility due to the exposure to excessive heat from malposition of the testes. Increased testicular temperature impairs the immature cells from transforming into sperm-producing cells. The transformation process happens early in life, between 3 and 8 months of age.[24] The best measure of male fertility is time to conception of a live born child, which involves multiple confounding variables, and need for long-term follow-up, making it challenging to quantify. Hence, measures such as testicular volume, histology, and semen analysis have been used as surrogates of testicular function.

In prepubertal boys, testicular volume on serial measurements correlates well to spermatogenic activity and adult testicular volume.[25] Testicular biopsy at the time of orchidopexy is currently not recommended because it may cause harm to the testis and the findings do not accurately predict fertility.[26]

Early surgical intervention for optimization of fertility surrogate measures is supported by the literature. Kollin and colleagues compared the growth of congenital unilateral UDT who were randomized to undergo orchidopexy at age 9 months versus 3 years and found improved testicular growth in the early orchidopexy group.[27]

Park and colleagues compared testicular histology in patients with unilateral UDT at the time of orchidopexy to age-matched children. They found mean tubular fertility index and germ cell count in patients aged 1 year or younger at the time of orchidopexy to be significantly higher than in children aged between 1 and 2 years and that these parameters were significantly worse in children greater than 2 at the time of surgery.[28] These studies and others support the recommendation that orchidopexy should be performed before 1 year of age to optimize fertility outcomes.[29]

Although the paternity of men with corrected nonsyndromic unilateral UDT is thought to be similar to the general population without UDT, 85% to 90% versus 90% to 92%, respectively, cryptorchidism is one of the most commonly reported comorbidities (17%) in men evaluated for infertility.[30,31] Patients with bilateral UDT tend to be at risk of infertility despite early orchidopexy, suggesting there is a global dysfunction of the testicles. Infertility in patients with bilateral UDT is estimated at 45% to 60%.[32]

Increased Risk of Testicular Cancer

The risk of developing testicular cancer in men with a history of UDT is 2 to 5-fold higher than the general population. The risk is reduced in patients who were diagnosed and treated before puberty. The proposed mechanism for the increased cancer risk is the lack of transformation of cells from juvenile gonocytes means cells persist in the undifferentiated form and are therefore more likely to undergo malignant transformation.[32]

A large cohort study observing nearly 17,000 Swedish patients who had an orchidopexy found higher than expected number of cases of testicular cancer with a relative risk (RR) of 2.23 (CI 95%, 1.58–3.06) compared with the general population and this increased to an RR of 5.40 (CI 95%, 3.20–8.53) for those treated at the age of 13 years or older.[33]

The Swedish Cancer Registry has compulsory reporting of all cancers. Trabert and colleagues identified cryptorchidism as an independent risk factor for testicular germ cell tumors with an OR of 3.16 (CI 95%, 2.45–3.96), higher than all other genital malformations.[34] In untreated UDT the primary pathologic condition is seminoma (74%), whereas nonseminomas are more prevalent in scrotal testes (63%).[35]

The best evidence suggests orchidopexy before puberty to reduce the risk of testicular cancer, and relocate the testis for easier self-examination. For postpubertal men with unilateral abdominal or hypotrophic UDT, orchiectomy may be a better option weighing the increased risk of testicular

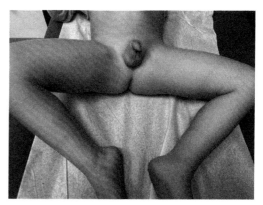

Fig. 2. A 2-year-old boy with left undescended testicle and scrotal asymmetry outlining optimal frog-legged positioning to enhance effectiveness of physical examination.

cancer and the functional benefit of performing an orchidopexy.

CLINICAL PRESENTATION AND DIAGNOSTIC APPROACH

The diagnosis of UDT is made clinically with genital physical examination by bimanual palpation with or without lubrication. The method for the testicular examination depends on the age of the child. For infants, the supine frog leg position (**Fig. 2**) or sitting in the parent's lap is ideal. To identify the lowest position of the testicle, examiners should place gentle downward pressure over the inguinal canal while palpating with the other hand. Older children may be examined in the supine position. In addition, the groin, femoral region, pubic area, and perineum should be palpated in search of an ectopic testis.[26] **Fig. 1** outlines the locations of true UDT and the possible ectopic locations of testicles.

There is No Role for Imaging in Detecting the Presence and Position of an UDT

Imaging modalities that have been investigated include ultrasound and MRI. However, the sensitivity and specificity of ultrasound for localizing an NPT is only 45% and 78%, respectively.[36] MRI performed slightly better with a sensitivity of 65% and specificity of 100%.[37] Additionally, MRI may necessitate sedation or general anesthesia in pediatric patients, which is not cost effective and confers additional risk. In a study of 169 boys referred for UDT, ultrasound only had a 34% concordance with the urologist's physical examination findings.[38]

Furthermore, imaging is inaccurate for diagnosing a vanishing or absent testis in those with NPT and does not eliminate the need for surgical confirmation. Specifically, if imaging identifies an intra-abdominal testis, surgery will remain necessary. In patients where imaging cannot identify a viable testis, an examination under anesthesia (EUA) will still be required and if there is no palpable testis, a diagnostic laparoscopy will be required. Therefore, imaging does not lead to a change in the management plan and may be associated with significant delays to accessing specialized surgical care.

Studies demonstrate that boys who underwent prereferral ultrasound wait longer to see a specialist and delays surgical correction.[39] Unnecessary imaging has additional impacts in resource limited health-care systems with important financial implications. Avoiding imaging for UDT is supported by Choosing Wisely Canada and multiple urological association guidelines due to diagnostic inaccuracies, delayed referral to specialists, and increased costs to the system.[26,40,41]

Although not perfect, clinical predictors of an absent viable testis have been described, such as size and location of the contralateral testicle and presence of hypoplastic hemiscrotum/scrotal asymmetry.[42] Testicular hypertrophy with a volume greater than 2 mL has been shown to be a significant predictor of monorchism with 71.7% sensitivity and 100% specificity.[43] However, testicular hypertrophy should not be used to forgo proper surgical exploration in the setting of an NPT, as leaving an unrecognized intra-abdominal testis could be associated with significant long-term morbidity.[44]

Pediatricians and primary care physicians should be educated about the expected timing of spontaneous descent (>90% by 3 months of age in full-term boys). Boys with UDT should be referred to a surgical specialist if the testicle remains undescended between 3 and 6 months (corrected for gestational age). The ideal age of surgical intervention based on published guidelines is 6 to 18 months.[26,41]

SPECIAL SITUATIONS

Patients with bilateral NPT should be referred for a DSD workup promptly due to the possibility of congenital adrenal hyperplasia (CAH) with complete virilization of the external genitalia. Although most of these patients will bear an XY karyotype and constitute males with bilateral UDT, the rare missed diagnosis of salt-wasting CAH is potentially catastrophic and associated with significant negative repercussions for the patient and the family.

Patients with bilateral NPT and XY karyotype should be evaluated for testicular regression syndrome, typically associated with low testosterone levels and high gonadotropin levels. Referral to an endocrinologist is recommended to evaluate for hormonal abnormalities and their consequences.[8,45] If levels of inhibin B and anti-Mullerian hormone are very low/undetectable, a clinical diagnosis of testes regression syndrome can be made and surgery may be avoided.

Patients presenting with proximal hypospadias and at least one UDT will be diagnosed with a DSD in up to 47% of cases.[46,47] Therefore, a DSD workup is recommended in this situation. Furthermore, WT1 testing is also warranted in this particular population and screening for Wilms tumor will be necessary in those who are found to carry the gene.

Finally, an UDT that is found intraoperatively to be attached to Mullerian structures, such as

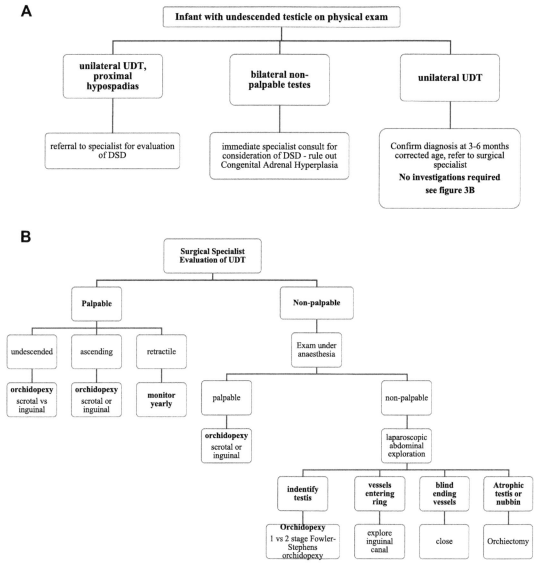

Fig. 3. (*A*) Basic algorithm for primary care physicians (PCP) identification of cryptorchidism and referral patterns. (*B*) Algorithm for surgical assessment and management of UDT.

remnants of the uterus or fallopian tubes, is indicative of Persistent Mullerian Duct syndrome. This is caused by an autosomal recessive genetic mutation.[48] Referral to endocrinology and measurements of serum anti-Mullerian hormone levels is recommended, along with surgical removal of the Mullerian remnants at the time of orchidopexy.

TREATMENT

The mainstay of treatment of UDT is surgical. Although medical therapies using human chorionic gonadotropin or luteinizing hormone-releasing hormone to facilitate descent are generally safe, they do not portray good efficacy and are rarely recommended.[49] The primary goals of surgical correction include optimization of testicular function and facilitation of examination for testicular masses. After referral to Urology for testes not within the normal scrotal position by 6 months, or bilateral UDT, surgical correction is recommended between 6 and 18 months of age as spontaneous descent is very unlikely and early orchidopexy is associated with better outcomes for testicular development.

Despite these age recommendations, multiple studies show the age of orchidopexy on average is actually much later.[50] One study performed in a single-payer health-care system reported 75% of orchidopexies for UDT occurs beyond

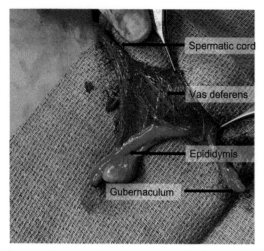

Fig. 4. Left inguinal orchidopexy with dashed lines showing pathway of long looping vas deferens. Highlights the importance of dividing the gubernaculum as distally as possible with the vas under direct vision.

18 months with the average age of 24 months, and age of first consult was 20 months. This suggests that the limiting factor for timely intervention is often late referrals.[51] Other identified factors that delay referral include normal testicular examination at birth, history of "retractile testis" and diagnosis not made by primary health-care provider.[50] Although multiple factors contribute to delayed surgeries, the general recommendation to improve the wait time for surgery is through improved educational efforts for primary care physicians.[51–53]

Fig. 3 outlines an algorithm for the detection of UDT, referral patterns, and surgical assessment and management.

SURGICAL TECHNIQUE
Palpable Testis

Inguinal approach
Traditionally, the palpable UDT, ectopic, or ascending testicle is approached through an inguinal incision. After dividing the external oblique fascia and delivering the testis, the gubernaculum is usually identified and divided. Attention should be paid to the insertion of the vas because some patients can present with a long looping vas that extends down away from the testicle and could be inadvertently damaged during this step (**Fig. 4**).

Attachments between the spermatic cord and the inguinal canal are dissected bluntly all the way to the internal inguinal ring; the key step to gain length and allow a tension-free orchidopexy is the dissection of the patent processus vaginalis from the cord, which can be tedious. The hernia sac tends to be very thin and separation from the cord is more difficult than what is typically encountered in a patient with a hydrocele or inguinal hernia. Additionally, it is important for the surgeon to be mindful of variants of anatomy including a long-looping vas deferens (see **Fig. 4**) or nonfusion of the epididymis.[54]

Dissection of the hernia sac
This can be accomplished through the usual anterior approach, where the antero-medial patent processus vaginalis is separated from the spermatic vessels and vas deferens. Because the hernia sac is often so thin, a breach is common and can lead to tears in the sac, which makes the dissection more difficult. Some surgeons deliberately open the hernia sac and dissect the cord structures from its posterior aspect under direct vision, placing several hemostats on the proximal

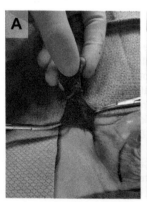
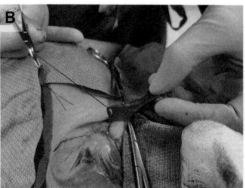
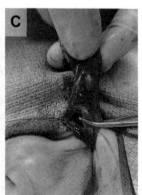

Fig. 5. Right prescrotal orchidopexy outlining posterior approach. (*A*) Hemostats exposing external spermatic fascia and patent processus vaginalis. (*B*) Suture tie surrounding cord structures dissected from patent processus vaginalis. (*C*) Hemostat placed across patent processus vaginalis before transection with cord structures protected and under direct visualization.

edges of the sac as dissection progresses (Clatworthy). Once the cord structures are free, the hernia sac is clamped making sure to include its full circumference and dissection continues to the level of the internal ring. Sufficient length can be achieved in the majority of cases for palpable testes with mobilization to this level. The hernia sac is suture ligated with an absorbable suture (Vicryl).

An alternative to the dissection of the hernia sac is the posterior approach, where the testicle is manually retracted upward and the cord structures are identified first. The vas and vessels are elevated from the hernia sac and protected with a small piece of suture or vessel loop for retraction. After confirming that the cord structures are safeguarded, the surgeon can clamp and divide the hernia sac. Dissection then proceeds toward the internal ring as previously described. The authors favor the posterior approach for palpable testes in most cases. **Fig. 5** outlines the intraoperative steps of the posterior approach.

Less commonly, dissection to the level of the internal ring is not enough for the testis to reach the scrotum without tension and extramobilization is required. In such cases, the surgeon can retract the processus vaginalis anteriorly and enter the retroperitoneum, where blunt dissection while keeping gentle downward traction on the testis can allow additional length to be gained. Transposing the testis underneath the epigastric vessels is a described maneuver (Prentiss) to reduce the distance between the gonad and the scrotum that can be used in selected cases.

Scrotal fixation
Once adequate mobilization has been achieved, a tunnel between the inguinal incision and the scrotum is created bluntly. A transverse scrotal incision is performed and a subdartos pouch is fashioned through blunt dissection. The testicle is delivered through the scrotal incision and the orchidopexy is performed. Some surgeons will use sutures between the tunica albuginea and the subdartos pouch to secure the testis, whereas others will simply place the testis in the pouch without any fixation if there is no tension.

Concern has been raised in the literature about potential harms associated with suture fixation, although the quality of these reports is low. The authors tend not to use stitches as long as there is good testicular/cord mobility; in such cases, placement of a stitch on either side of the cord through the spermatic fascia after transposing

the testis to make the neck of the opening snug prevents reascension.

Prescrotal approach
In the last few years, the single incision, prescrotal approach described by Bianchi has gained popularity.[55,56] In this technique, the orchidopexy is performed with a single incision on the lateral aspect of the scrotum on the affected side. Although some surgeons advocate for the prescrotal approach for every palpable testis, others suggest that it should be reserved for testes in a lower, closer to the scrotum position. The authors tend to favor the prescrotal approach for testes palpable below the level of the external inguinal ring.

After performing the prescrotal incision, the subdartos pouch is created. Systematic use of retraction to identify the testis allows it to be delivered through the incision in a similar fashion to the inguinal approach. Gubernacular attachments and adhesions to the inguinal canal and external ring are released. Cephalad retraction right on the spermatic cord allows a high ligation of the hernia sac to be performed. Dissection of the hernia sac follows the same principles described before for the inguinal approach; the posterior approach to the hernia sac is also feasible with the prescrotal incision.

Nonpalpable testis
As mentioned previously, there is no role for imaging in the management of the NPT. Patients aged older than 6 months with an NPT should be booked for a surgical intervention; **Fig. 3B** illustrates the algorithm used to approach boys with an NPT once in the operating room. By following the steps described, the presence of viable

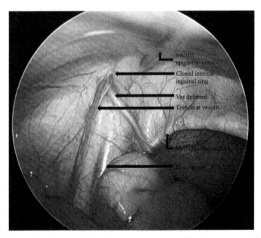

Fig. 6. Diagnostic laparoscopy outlining normal anatomy.

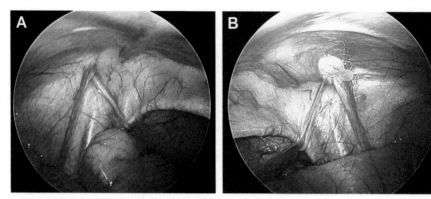

Fig. 7. Diagnostic laparoscopy findings for nonpalpable undescended testicle. (*A*) Left internal inguinal ring closed with normal testicular vessels and vas deferens. This could be compatible with a normal inguinal testis or a vanishing testis. Inguinal exploration is indicated. (*B*) Peeping right testicle with open internal inguinal ring and normal vas and vessels.

testicular tissue and its location can be ascertained with certainty that approaches 100%.

In summary, after induction an EUA is performed. Up to 20% of testes that were not detectable in the office setting will be palpated in the operating room when the child is fully relaxed.[57] The surgeon can then proceed with an inguinal orchidopexy. If the testis remains nonpalpable, a diagnostic laparoscopy is the next step.

The normal anatomy of the closed internal inguinal ring is shown in **Fig. 6**. The intraoperative findings of a left testicle that is descended, and shows normal closed internal ring anatomy is shown in **Fig. 7**A and a right "peeping" intra-abdominal testicle in **Fig. 7**B. It is important to keep in mind the embryological association of the testis with the testicular vessels rather than the vas deferens. Hence, the observation of blind ending testicular vessels confirms the diagnosis of anorchia, whereas a testis may still be present in a patient diagnosed with a blind-ending vas.

Visualization of the vas and vessels traversing the internal inguinal ring in the absence of a palpable inguinal gonad suggests the diagnosis of a vanishing testis, that is, a nonviable nubbin that was probably the subject of a torsion or other ischemic event in utero. Most urologists will go ahead with an inguinal or prescrotal exploration in this situation to remove the nubbin, although the pathology literature has shown that the presence of viable germ cells in these cases is quite rare.[58,59]

Diagnostic laparoscopy will confirm the presence of an intra-abdominal testis in approximately 50% of cases.[60] The testicle can be found anywhere between a high retroperitoneal location close to the lower pole of the kidney to a "peeping" position at the level of the internal inguinal ring. In certain cases where there is adequate testicular mobility in the setting of an intra-abdominal testicle, a primary laparoscopic orchidopexy can be completed. **Fig. 8** outlines intraoperative images of a primary laparoscopic orchidopexy.

High intra-abdominal testes can be challenging to mobilize into the scrotum, usually due to insufficient vessel length. A modification of the traditional Fowler-Stephens orchidopexy was developed into a 2-stage approach where the gonadal vessels are clipped laparoscopically in the first stage. The orchidopexy is then completed (open or laparoscopic) approximately 6 months later in a second stage.[61,62] If there is a patent processus vaginalis, the surgeon can use that to bring the testis down sparing the gubernaculum, which can preserve additional blood supply.[63,64] If the processus vaginalis is closed, a new path is created with a trocar under direct visualization, usually between the bladder and the obliterated umbilical artery (median ligament).

The choice of technique and outcomes of orchidopexy for intra-abdominal testes hinges mostly on a high versus low abdominal position. A study comparing outcomes of 64 NPT where a 2-staged Fowler-Stephens approach was selected for high abdominal position and a primary orchidopexy for low abdominal position found good outcomes in each group. At the time of follow-up, all patients in the orchidopexy and low testicular position group (n = 28) had orthotopic testicles and no evidence of atrophy, whereas the Fowler-Stephens group with high position had an overall success rate of 88.8%, with 2 cases of testicular displacement and 2 cases of testicular atrophy on follow-up.[65]

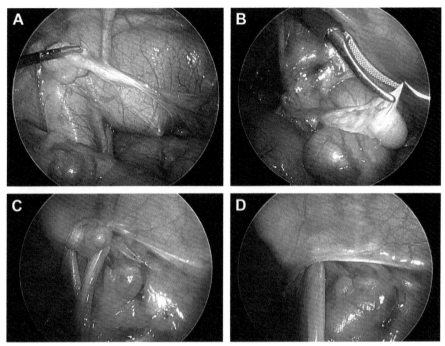

Fig. 8. Steps of a right primary laparoscopic orchidopexy. (*A*) Right testicle is dissected fully from peritoneum and mobilized to contralateral internal inguinal ring depicting adequate length. (*B*) Trocar advanced from scrotum to peritoneum via inguinal canal and right testicle secured to Maryland grasper. (*C*) Testicle, along with grasper and trocar, are brought down to scrotum via inguinal canal. (*D*) Testicular vessels descending through the inguinal canal.

SURGICAL OUTCOMES

Successful orchidopexy is typically defined as a normal scrotal position and absence of testicular atrophy. Other considerations for selecting the optimal surgical approach include minimizing short-term complications such as infection, hematoma, wound dehiscence, and pain.

A meta-analysis comparing orchidopexy outcomes in a total of 2627 children with palpable UDT for both open scrotal and open inguinal approaches reported testicular atrophy occurred in 0.6% to 0.9% (OR 0.64, 95% CI 0.27–1.53) of cases, and testicular reascent in about 2.0% (OR 1.06, 95% CI 0.62–1.79) with no significant difference between the 2 approaches.[66]

A randomized control trial comparing inguinal to scrotal orchidopexy in 161 patients found 3 patients had testicular reascent and 1 patient had testicular atrophy, with all these complications occurring in the scrotal approach group.[67] Both procedures were associated with low postoperative pain; however, the scrotal approach was associated with lower pain scores.[67] Orchidopexy for palpable UDT has excellent overall success with a low rate of complications. Conversely, the success rates for correction of NPT are lower

than for palpable UDT, ranging from 63% to 97%.[68,69]

There is no consensus around the best technique to manage the intra-abdominal testis. A few published systematic reviews favor the staged approach,[61,70] whereas others fail to identify a clear advantage of 1-stage versus 2-stage Fowler-Stephens orchidopexy.[49,71] Most included studies in these reviews are single-institution case series and no robust clinical trials have been conducted to date. The exact position of the testis at the start of treatment needs to be properly ascertained to allow a fair comparison between techniques.

Recently, a technique has been described where the vessels are not clipped, even for high intra-abdominal testes. After extensive laparoscopic mobilization, the testis is secured to the abdominal wall immediately above and medial to the contralateral anterior superior iliac spine (Shehata technique).[72] After 12 weeks, the testis is again mobilized laparoscopically and able to reach the scrotum without division of the vessels. Some authors have demonstrated enthusiasm with this technique but experience is still limited compared with the others described.[49,73] The choice of surgical management for the high intra-abdominal testis would benefit from a well-designed clinical trial.

CLINICS CARE POINTS

- Undescended testicles should undergo surgical treatment between 6 and 18 months of age.
- Imaging does not change management in boys with nonpalpable testes and may result is delays to surgical treatment.
- The presence of bilateral nonpalpable gonads should raise the suspicion for DSD. A diagnostic workup should be performed before embarking on surgical treatment.

DISCLOSURE

The authors have no financial or commercial conflicts of interest to disclose. This study did not receive any external funding.

REFERENCES

1. Wohlfahrt-Veje C, Boisen KA, Boas M, et al. Acquired cryptorchidism is frequent in infancy and childhood. Int J Androl 2009;32(4):423–8.
2. Hutson JM, Li R, Southwell BR, et al. Regulation of testicular descent. Pediatr Surg Int 2015;31(4):317–25.
3. Hutson JM, Nation T, Balic A, et al. Therapeutic Advances in Urology The role of the gubernaculum in the descent and undescent of the testis. Ther Adv Urol 2009;1(2):115–21.
4. Barthold JS, Reinhardt S, Thorup J. Genetic, Maternal, and Environmental Risk Factors for Cryptorchidism: An Update. Eur J Pediatr Surg 2016;26(5):399–408.
5. Acerini CL, Miles HL, Dunger DB, et al. The descriptive epidemiology of congenital and acquired cryptorchidism in a UK infant cohort. Arch Dis Child 2009;94(11):868–72.
6. Stec AA, Thomas JC, DeMarco RT, et al. Incidence of testicular ascent in boys with retractile testes. J Urol 2007;178(4 Pt 2):1722–5.
7. Gadelkareem RA, Shahat AA, Reda A, et al. Ectopic testis: an experience of a tertiary-level urology center at Upper Egypt. Annals of Pediatric Surgery 2020;16(1):1–9.
8. Elamo HP, Virtanen HE, Toppari J. Genetics of cryptorchidism and testicular regression. Best Pract Res Clin Endocrinol Metab 2022;36(1). https://doi.org/10.1016/J.BEEM.2022.101619.
9. Sijstermans K, Hack WWM, Meijer RW, et al. The frequency of undescended testis from birth to adulthood: A review. Int J Androl 2008;31(1):1–11.
10. Boisen KA, Kaleva M, Main KM, et al. Difference in prevalence of congenital cryptorchidism in infants between two Nordic countries. Lancet 2004;363(9417):1264–9.
11. Wagner-Mahler K, Kurzenne JY, Delattre I, et al. Prospective study on the prevalence and associated risk factors of cryptorchidism in 6246 newborn boys from Nice area, France. Int J Androl 2011;34(5 Pt 2). https://doi.org/10.1111/J.1365-2605.2011.01211.X.
12. Cendron M, Huff DS, Keating MA, et al. Anatomical, morphological and volumetric analysis: a review of 759 cases of testicular maldescent. J Urol 1993;149(3):570–3.
13. Lane C, Boxall J, MacLellan D, et al. A population-based study of prevalence trends and geospatial analysis of hypospadias and cryptorchidism compared with non-endocrine mediated congenital anomalies. J Pediatr Urol 2017;13(3):284.e1–7.
14. Mahboubi K, MacDonald L, Ahrens B, et al. Geospatial analysis of hypospadias and cryptorchidism prevalence rates based on postal code in a Canadian province with stable population. J Pediatr Urol 2023;19(1). https://doi.org/10.1016/J.JPUROL.2022.09.017.
15. Leslie SW, Sajjad H, Villanueva CA. Cryptorchidism. StatPearls. Published online November 28, 2022. Available at: https://www.ncbi.nlm.nih.gov/books/NBK470270/. Accessed February 24, 2023.
16. Ö Pirgon, Dündar BN. Vanishing Testes: A Literature Review. J Clin Res Pediatr Endocrinol 2012;4(3):116.
17. Baker LA, Docimo SG, Surer I, et al. A multi-institutional analysis of laparoscopic orchidopexy. BJU Int 2001;87(6):484–9.
18. Inan M, Aydiner CY, Tokuc B, et al. Prevalence of cryptorchidism, retractile testis and orchiopexy in school children. Urol Int 2008;80(2):166–71.
19. Van Brakel J, Kranse R, De Muinck Keizer-Schrama SMPF, et al. Fertility potential in a cohort of 65 men with previously acquired undescended testes. J Pediatr Surg 2014;49(4):599–605.
20. Meij-Devries A, Van Der Voort LM, Sijstermans K, et al. Natural course of undescended testes after inguinoscrotal surgery. J Pediatr Surg 2013;48(12):2540–4.
21. Herzog B, Steigert M, Hadziselimovic F. Is a Testis Located at the Superficial Inguinal Pouch (Denis Browne Pouch) Comparable to a True Cryptorchid Testis? J Urol 1992;148(2):622–3.
22. Hutcheson JC, Snyder HM, Zuñiga ZV, et al. Ectopic and undescended testes: 2 variants of a single congenital anomaly? J Urol 2000;163(3):961–3.
23. Celayir AC, Sander S, Eliçevik M. Timing of surgery in perineal ectopic testes: analysis of 16 cases. Pediatr Surg Int 2001;17(2–3):167–8.

24. Ong C, Hasthorpe S, Hutson JM. Germ cell development in the descended and cryptorchid testis and the effects of hormonal manipulation. Pediatr Surg Int 2005;21(4):240–54.

25. Takihara H, Cosentino MJ, Sakatoku J, et al. Significance of testicular size measurement in andrology: II. Correlation of testicular size with testicular function. J Urol 1987;137(3):416–9.

26. Evaluation and Treatment of Cryptorchidism (2018) - American Urological Association. Availabl e at: https://www.auanet.org/guidelines-and-quality/guidelines/cryptorchidism-guideline. Accessed March 7, 2023.

27. Kollin C, Hesser U, Ritzén EM, et al. Testicular growth from birth to two years of age, and the effect of orchidopexy at age nine months: a randomized, controlled study. Acta Paediatr 2006;95(3):318–24.

28. Park KH, Lee JH, Han JJ, et al. Histological evidences suggest recommending orchiopexy within the first year of life for children with unilateral inguinal cryptorchid testis. Int J Urol 2007;14(7):616–21.

29. Chan E, Wayne C, Nasr A. Ideal timing of orchiopexy: a systematic review. Pediatr Surg Int 2014;30(1):87–97.

30. Lee PA. Fertility after cryptorchidism: epidemiology and other outcome studies. Urology 2005;66(2):427–31.

31. Olesen IA, Andersson AM, Aksglaede L, et al. Clinical, genetic, biochemical, and testicular biopsy findings among 1,213 men evaluated for infertility. Fertil Steril 2017;107(1):74–82.e7.

32. Husmann DA. Cryptorchidism: What Are the Risks of Infertility? What Do We Tell the Parents? How Do We Manage the Child? J Urol 2022;207(3):498–9.

33. Pettersson A, Richiardi L, Nordenskjold A, et al. Age at surgery for undescended testis and risk of testicular cancer. N Engl J Med 2007;356(18):1835–41.

34. Trabert B, Zugna D, Richiardi L, et al. Congenital malformations and testicular germ cell tumors. Int J Cancer 2013;133(8):1900–4.

35. Wood HM, Lee UJ, Vurbic D, et al. Sexual development and fertility of Loxl1-/- male mice. J Androl 2009;30(4):452–9.

36. Tasian GE, Copp HL, Baskin LS. Diagnostic imaging in cryptorchidism: utility, indications, and effectiveness. J Pediatr Surg 2011;46(12):2406–13.

37. Krishnaswami S, Fonnesbeck C, Penson D, et al. Magnetic resonance imaging for locating nonpalpable undescended testicles: a meta-analysis. Pediatrics 2013;131(6). https://doi.org/10.1542/PEDS.2013-0073.

38. Wong NC, Bansal RK, Lorenzo AJ, et al. Misuse of ultrasound for palpable undescended testis by primary care providers: A prospective study. Can Urol Assoc J 2015;9(11–12):387–90.

39. Kanaroglou N, To T, Zhub J, et al. Inappropriate Use of Ultrasound in Management of Pediatric Cryptorchidism. Pediatrics 2015;136(3):479–86.

40. Urological Association C, Wisely Canada C. Urology Five Things Clinicians and Patients Should Question by Canadian Urological Association. Published online 2013. Available at: www.americangeriatrics.org. Accessed March 7, 2023.

41. Braga LH, Lorenzo AJ, Romao RLP. Canadian Urological Association-Pediatric Urologists of Canada (CUA-PUC) guideline for the diagnosis, management, and followup of cryptorchidism. Canadian Urological Association Journal 2017;11(7):E251.

42. Snodgrass W, Bush N, Holzer M, et al. Current referral patterns and means to improve accuracy in diagnosis of undescended testis. Pediatrics 2011;127(2). https://doi.org/10.1542/PEDS.2010-1719.

43. Hodhod A, Capolicchio JP, Jednak R, et al. Testicular hypertrophy as a predictor for contralateral monorchism: Retrospective review of prospectively recorded data. J Pediatr Urol 2016;12(1):34.e1–5.

44. Wei Y, Yu C, Zhou Y, et al. Testicular hypertrophy as predictor of contralateral nonpalpable testis among Chinese boys: An 18-year retrospective study. Arch Pediatr 2020;27(8):456–63.

45. Heksch RA, Matheson MA, Tishelman AC, et al. Testicular regression syndrome: practice variation in diagnosis and management. Endocr Pract 2019;25(8):779–86.

46. Cox MJ, Coplen DE, Austin PF. The Incidence of Disorders of Sexual Differentiation and Chromosomal Abnormalities of Cryptorchidism and Hypospadias Stratified by Meatal Location. J Urol 2008;180(6):2649–52.

47. Sekaran P, O'Toole S, Flett M, et al. Increased occurrence of disorders of sex development, prematurity and intrauterine growth restriction in children with proximal hypospadias associated with undescended testes. J Urol 2013;189(5):1892–6.

48. Picard JY, Cate RL, Racine C, et al. The Persistent Müllerian Duct Syndrome: An Update Based Upon a Personal Experience of 157 Cases. Sex Dev 2017;11(3):109–25.

49. Gates RL, Shelton J, Diefenbach KA, et al. Management of the undescended testis in children: An American Pediatric Surgical Association Outcomes and Evidence Based Practice Committee Systematic Review. J Pediatr Surg 2022;57(7):1293–308.

50. Jiang DD, Acevedo AM, Bayne A, et al. Factors associated with delay in undescended testis referral. J Pediatr Urol 2019;15(4):380.e1–6.

51. Dave S, Clark J, Chan EP, et al. Factors which delay surgery for undescended testis in Ontario: A retrospective population based cohort study on timing of orchidopexy between 2006 and 2012. J Pediatr Urol 2022;18(5):695.e1–7.

52. Boehme P, Degener S, Wirth S, et al. Multicenter Analysis of Acquired Undescended Testis and Its Impact on the Timing of Orchidopexy. J Pediatr 2020;223:170–7.e3.

53. Brown JJ, Wacogne I, Fleckney S, et al. Achieving early surgery for undescended testes: quality improvement through a multifaceted approach to guideline implementation. Child Care Health Dev 2004;30(2):97–102.

54. Kim SO, Na SW, Yu HS, et al. Epididymal anomalies in boys with undescended testis or hydrocele: Significance of testicular location. BMC Urol 2015;15(1). https://doi.org/10.1186/S12894-015-0099-1.

55. Bianchi A. Squire BR. Transscrotal orchidopexy: orchidopexy revised. Pediatr Surg Int 1989;4(3):189–92.

56. Dayanc M, Kibar Y, Irkilata HC, et al. Long-term outcome of scrotal incision orchiopexy for undescended testis. Urology 2007;70(4):786–8.

57. Cisek LJ, Peters CA, Atala A, et al. Current findings in diagnostic laparoscopic evaluation of the non-palpable testis. J Urol 1998;160(3 Pt 2):1145–9.

58. Woodford E, Eliezer D, Deshpande A, et al. Is excision of testicular nubbin necessary in vanishing testis syndrome? J Pediatr Surg 2018;53(12):2495–7.

59. Nataraja RM, Asher CM, Nash R, et al. Is routine excision of testicular remnants in testicular regression syndrome indicated? J Pediatr Urol 2015;11(3):151.e1.

60. Elder JS. Surgical Management of the Undescended Testis: Recent Advances and Controversies. Eur J Pediatr Surg 2016;26(5):418–26.

61. Elyas R, Guerra LA, Pike J, et al. Is staging beneficial for Fowler-Stephens orchiopexy? A systematic review. J Urol 2010;183(5):2012–9.

62. Ransley PG, Vordermark JS, Caldamone AA, et al. Preliminary ligation of the gonadal vessels prior to orchidopexy for the intra-abdominal testicle - A staged Fowler-Stephens procedure. World J Urol 1984;2(4):266–8.

63. Robertson SA, Munro FD, MacKinlay GA. Two-stage Fowler-Stephens orchidopexy preserving the gubernacular vessels and a purely laparoscopic second stage. J Laparoendosc Adv Surg Tech 2007;17(1):101–7.

64. Braga LH, Farrokhyar F, McGrath M, et al. Gubernaculum Testis and Cremasteric Vessel Preservation during Laparoscopic Orchiopexy for Intra-Abdominal Testes: Effect on Testicular Atrophy Rates. J Urol 2019;201(2):378–85.

65. Moursy EE, Gamal W, Hussein MM. Laparoscopic orchiopexy for non-palpable testes: outcome of two techniques. J Pediatr Urol 2011;7(2):178–81.

66. Yu C, Hu Y, Wang L, et al. Comparison of Single-Incision Scrotal Orchiopexy and Traditional Two-Incision Inguinal Orchiopexy for Primary Palpable Undescended Testis in Children: A Systematic Review and Meta-Analysis. Front Pediatr 2022;10. https://doi.org/10.3389/FPED.2022.805579.

67. McGrath M, Kim J, Farrokhyar F, et al. Randomized Controlled Trial of Scrotal versus Inguinal Orchidopexy on Postoperative Pain. J Urol 2021;205(3):895–901.

68. Docimo SG, Moore RG, Adams J, et al. Laparoscopic Orchiopexy for High Palpable Undescended Testis: Preliminary Experience. J Urol 1995;154(4):1513–5.

69. Stec AA, Tanaka ST, Adams MC, et al. Orchiopexy for intra-abdominal testes: factors predicting success. J Urol 2009;182(4 Suppl):1917–20.

70. Yu C, Long C, Wei Y, et al. Evaluation of Fowler-Stephens orchiopexy for high-level intra-abdominal cryptorchidism: A systematic review and meta-analysis. Int J Surg 2018;60:74–87.

71. Wayne C, Chan E, Nasr A. What is the ideal surgical approach for intra-abdominal testes? a systematic review. Pediatr Surg Int 2015;31(4):327–38.

72. Shehata S, Shalaby R, Ismail M, et al. Staged laparoscopic traction-orchiopexy for intraabdominal testis (Shehata technique) Stretching the limits for preservation of testicular vasculature. J Pediatr Surg 2016;51(2):211–5.

73. Qingqing T, Xiang Z, Chu Z, et al. Compared outcomes of high-level cryptorchidism managed by Fowler-Stephens orchiopexy versus the Shehata technique: A systematic review and meta-analysis. J Pediatr Urol 2023. https://doi.org/10.1016/J.JPUROL.2023.02.025.